THE NO GALLBLADDER DIET COOKBOOK FOR BEGINNERS 2024

Delicious Low-Fat Recipes and Expert Tips for optimal digestion, Metabolic Balance, and Post-Surgery Vitality with a 90-day nutritious meal plan.

Carol Troxel

TABLE OF CONTENTS

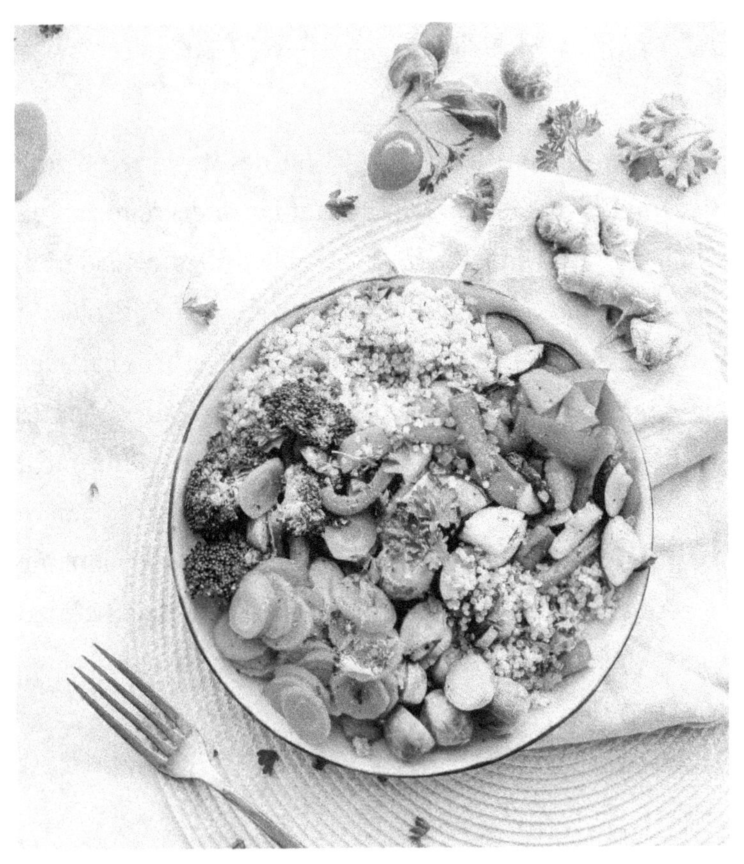

INTRODUCTION

Welcome to your brand-new journey toward healthy digestion, metabolic equilibrium, and rejuvenated vitality! If you are reading this, all things considered, you or a friend or family member has gone through a gallbladder evacuation medical procedure. This can be a big change, but it also means the start of a new chapter with opportunities to adopt healthier eating habits and a more mindful nutrition approach. Whether you're recently presented with a medical procedure or looking to refine your eating routine for better stomach-related well-being, this book is here to direct you constantly.

Understanding Life Without a Gallbladder

Living without a gallbladder could appear to be overwhelming from the start, yet with the right information and devices, you can flourish. The gallbladder assumes a part in processing by putting away bile, which helps separate fats. Your body will adjust without it by sending bile directly to the small intestine from the liver. This truly means that while you can partake in various food varieties, it's critical to be aware of fat admission and what various food varieties mean for your absorption.

You may experience changes in your digestive patterns and tolerance to certain foods. Some might find that high-fat or greasy meals cause discomfort, while others might notice a difference in how their body responds to dairy or spicy foods. The key is to listen to your body and adapt accordingly. This book is designed to help you navigate these changes confidently, offering a wealth of delicious, low-fat recipes that support your digestive health and overall well-being.

How to Use This Book

"The Complete No Gallbladder Diet Cookbook for Beginners 2024" is structured to provide you with everything you need to succeed on this journey. Here's how to make the most of it:

- Educational Insights: Start with the chapters that explain the function of the gallbladder, the reasons for its removal, and the digestive changes you can expect. You'll be able to make better food choices if you know these fundamentals.

- Nutritional Guidelines: Learn about the essential nutrients and food groups that support optimal digestion. Discover which foods to embrace and which to avoid, along with tips for maintaining a balanced and satisfying diet.

- Recipes: Dive into a wide array of recipes, carefully crafted to be low in fat and high in flavor. From breakfast to dinner, snacks to desserts, you'll find options that cater to every taste and occasion. Each recipe includes nutritional information to help you keep track of your intake.

- 90-Day Meal Plan: To make your transition smoother, we've included a 90-day meal plan complete with shopping lists and meal prep tips. This plan is designed to take the guesswork out of your daily meals and ensure you're nourishing your body with wholesome, delicious foods.

- Expert Tip: Benefit from tips on how to stay on track and long-term eating habits. These insights will offer practical tips and inspiration to keep you motivated.

By the end of this book, you'll not only have a collection of go-to recipes but also a more profound comprehension of your body's requirements and how to meet them.. Embrace this journey with an open heart and a positive mindset. Here's to a healthier, happier you!

CHAPTER 1:
UNDERSTANDING GALLBLADDER REMOVAL

The Gallbladder and Its Function

The gallbladder, a little pear-formed organ situated underneath the liver, assumes a vital part in the stomach-related framework. Notwithstanding its humble size, it has a critical capability: putting away and concentrating bile delivered by the liver. The digestion and absorption of dietary fats depend on bile, a digestive fluid. Understanding the gallbladder's capability gives knowledge into the stomach-related difficulties and changes one could look after its expulsion. Bile creation is ceaseless in the liver, however its emission into the small digestive system is managed. In response to food intake, particularly of fatty foods, the gallbladder releases bile as a reservoir. The gallbladder contracts when you eat, pushing bile into the small intestine through the bile ducts. Here, bile separates fats into smaller droplets that enzymes can further digest by emulsifying. This cycle is fundamental for the ingestion of fat-solvent nutrients (A, D, E, and K) and different supplements. Additionally, the gallbladder's bile concentration is crucial. The gallbladder stores and concentrates the bile that the liver continuously secretes by absorbing water and electrolytes. This concentrated bile is more successful in processing fats contrasted with the weakened bile that streams straightforwardly from the liver to the small digestive tract without a trace of the gallbladder. While the gallbladder isn't basic, its nonappearance requires changes in the stomach-related process. Without the gallbladder, bile streams straightforwardly from the liver into the small digestive tract at an increasingly slow focused rate. This modification may have an effect on how well fat is broken down, which could cause problems with malabsorption or discomfort in the digestive tract. The comprehension of the gallbladder's capability highlights the requirement for dietary changes post-evacuation. Low-fat meals help make up for the slower rate at which fat is digested. It's even more important to include foods high in fat-soluble vitamins and ensure a healthy balance of nutrients. With this information, one can more readily value the dietary rules and way of life changes suggested after gallbladder expulsion, guaranteeing smoother progress and ideal stomach-related well-being.

Reasons for Gallbladder Removal

Cholecystectomy, or removal of the gallbladder, is a common surgical procedure that is frequently required by various disorders or dysfunctions of the gallbladder. The choice to eliminate the gallbladder regularly comes from conditions that cause critical agony, contamination, or other serious well-being gambles. Gallstones (cholelithiasis) are a major reason for gallbladder removal. The gallbladder's bile cholesterol and bilirubin lead to the formation of gallstones, which are solid particles. They can differ in size and number, and keeping in mind that a few people might have gallstones without side effects, others can encounter serious torment, irritation, and contamination. At the point when gallstones block the bile channels, they can cause extreme agony known as biliary colic, as well as additional serious difficulties like intense cholecystitis (aggravation of the gallbladder), pancreatitis (irritation of the pancreas), or cholangitis (contamination of the bile pipes). In these cases, gallbladder evacuation is many times the best treatment to forestall repetitive episodes and serious well-being gambles. Gallbladder polyps are another reason to remove the gallbladder. These are growths that stick out of the gallbladder's lining. Although the majority of gallbladder polyps are benign and asymptomatic, larger polyps or those that cause symptoms may necessitate gallbladder removal to reduce the risk of gallbladder cancer. Another condition that calls for surgery is chronic cholecystitis or a disease of the gallbladder. This condition involves persistent gallbladder inflammation, which is frequently brought on by recurrent episodes of acute inflammation or gallstones. The gallbladder wall can become scarred and thickened as a result of chronic cholecystitis, reducing its functionality and resulting in persistent discomfort and digestive issues. The removal of the gallbladder has the potential to alleviate symptoms and prevent additional complications. For biliary dyskinesia, a condition characterized by a gallbladder that does not properly empty bile, gallbladder removal may be recommended in some instances. This brokenness can cause biliary colic even without a trace of gallstones. Gallbladder function can be evaluated using diagnostic tests like a HIDA scan, and if significant dysfunction is found, cholecystectomy can alleviate symptoms. In uncommon occurrences, gallbladder evacuation might be important because of gallbladder disease. Although gallbladder malignant growth is remarkable, it is normally identified at a late stage because of its asymptomatic nature in the beginning phases. Surgery to remove the gallbladder and stop cancer from spreading to other parts of the body is frequently required after a diagnosis. Generally, the choice to eliminate the gallbladder depends on an exhaustive assessment of side effects, symptomatic tests, and the expected dangers and advantages of a medical procedure. The objective is to reduce torment, forestall confusion, and work on personal satisfaction. Patients can better prepare for the lifestyle changes that come with gallbladder removal if they are aware of the reasons behind it.

Changes in Digestion Post-Surgery

Gallbladder expulsion, while lightening the side effects and dangers related to gallbladder infection, acquaints changes with the stomach-related process that requires cautious administration. Understanding these progressions is significant for adjusting to existence without a gallbladder and keeping up with ideal stomach-related well-being. Bile produced by the liver flows directly into the small intestine in a continuous, less concentrated stream when there is no gallbladder. The digestion and absorption of dietary fats, which are typically emulsified by bile during digestion, may be affected by this continuous flow. As a result, some people may have trouble digesting foods high in fat, which can cause symptoms like gas, bloating, diarrhea, and pain in the abdomen. These side effects, frequently alluded to as post-cholecystectomy disorder, can fluctuate in seriousness and length among people. One of the essential changes in absorption post-medical procedure is the decreased productivity in separating fats. It is possible that bile may not be as effective at simultaneously emulsifying large quantities of dietary fat because it is less concentrated and continuously present in the intestine. This can bring about fat malabsorption, where undigested fats go through the intestinal system, causing diarrheas or the runs. To moderate these impacts, an eating routine low in fat is suggested. Lean proteins, whole grains, fruits, and vegetables can support digestive health and help manage symptoms. Moreover, the modified bile stream can influence the stomach microbiome, the local area of useful microorganisms in the digestive organs. The balance of gut bacteria can be affected by changes in bile flow and composition, which may result in digestive issues. Foods high in probiotics and prebiotics, like yogurt, kefir, and fruits and vegetables high in fiber, can help maintain a healthy gut microbiome and improve digestion. Another thought is the effect on the ingestion of fat-solvent nutrients (A, D, E, and K). Since the flow of bile is continuous but less concentrated, there may be a chance that these vitamins won't be absorbed properly. Including these vitamins in a well-balanced diet or taking supplements under the supervision of a doctor can help prevent deficiencies and support overall health. Mindful eating is another aspect of post-surgery digestion management. The digestive system can handle food more efficiently if smaller, more frequent meals are consumed instead of large, bulky meals. Eating slowly and thoroughly can help digestion and lower the likelihood of discomfort. Remaining hydrated and integrating dissolvable fiber can likewise uphold sound processing and forestall stoppage. Now and again, people might encounter changes in entrail propensities, like expanded recurrence or direness. Changing your fiber intake, staying hydrated, and avoiding foods that cause symptoms are all ways to manage this. Keeping a food journal to follow feasts and side effects can assist with distinguishing explicit triggers and making vital changes. The majority of people find that their digestive system adapts over time, despite the challenging initial adjustment period following gallbladder removal. By embracing a fair, low-fat eating regimen and careful dietary patterns, it is feasible to oversee side effects and partake in a solid, dynamic way of life. It is also possible to ensure that any issues that persist are addressed and that overall health is maintained through regular follow-ups with healthcare providers. In conclusion, individuals are empowered to take proactive measures to manage their health by comprehending the changes in digestion following surgery. It is possible to successfully navigate life without a gallbladder and maintain optimal digestive and overall health with the right dietary choices and lifestyle adjustments.

CHAPTER 2:

ESSENTIAL NUTRITIONAL GUIDELINES

Key Nutrients for Optimal Digestion

A well-balanced intake of essential nutrients that help the digestive system function is necessary for optimal digestion. Concentrating on these nutrients is even more important for people who don't have a gallbladder to ensure that nutrients are absorbed and that digestion goes smoothly. One of the most essential nutrients for digestion is fiber. It comes in two structures: solvent and insoluble. In water, soluble fiber forms a gel-like substance that aids blood sugar and cholesterol management. It additionally eases back assimilation, taking into consideration better supplement ingestion and more continuous energy discharge. On the other hand, insoluble fiber makes the stool bulkier and helps food move through the digestive system, preventing constipation. Whole grains, nuts, legumes, and fruits are all sources of fiber. Integrating various food sources into your eating routine can advance ordinary solid discharges and generally speaking stomach stomach-related well-being. For optimal digestion, prebiotics and probiotics are also necessary. A healthy gut microbiome is essential for breaking down food, absorbing nutrients, and defending against harmful microorganisms. Probiotics are beneficial bacteria that assist in maintaining this healthy microbiome. Fibers called prebiotics feed these good bacteria and help them grow and do their jobs. Aged food sources like yogurt, kefir, sauerkraut, and kimchi are phenomenal wellsprings of probiotics, while prebiotics can be found in food sources like garlic, onions, bananas, and entire grains. Another crucial aspect of digestive health is staying hydrated. Water is essential for the processing and retention of supplements, as well as concerning the end of side effects. It helps break down dissolvable fiber, permitting it to go all the more effectively through the intestinal system, and forestalls stoppage by relaxing stool. If you are physically active or live in a hot climate, aim for eight glasses of water per day or more. The body naturally produces digestive enzymes to break down food into nutrients that can be absorbed. Amylase for carbohydrates, protease for proteins, and lipase for fats are examples of these. After gallbladder expulsion, the body's capacity to process fats productively can be compromised because of the nonstop however less focused progression of bile. Consolidating chemical-rich food sources like pineapples (bromelain), papayas (papain), and matured food varieties can help with absorption. A digestive enzyme supplement may also be beneficial in some instances; however, before beginning any supplementation, it is essential to consult a healthcare professional. You can support the health and functionality of your digestive system by focusing on these essential nutrients—fiber, probiotics, prebiotics, hydration, digestive enzymes—to ensure smoother digestion and improved nutrient absorption.

Low-Fat Diet Essentials

For people who do not have a gallbladder, a low-fat diet is essential because it helps control the decreased efficiency of fat digestion and prevents discomfort in the digestive tract. In addition to eliminating obvious fat sources, a low-fat diet necessitates a comprehensive understanding of food choices and preparation techniques that support digestive health. Begin by picking lean protein sources. These incorporate poultry without the skin, fish, beans, lentils, and tofu. Healthy omega-3 fatty acids are found in fish, particularly fatty fish like salmon and mackerel. These fatty acids are easier to digest and have anti-inflammatory properties. However, due to their fat content, these should be consumed in moderation. Even though eggs can be included, the yolks should be limited or avoided if they cause digestive issues due to their higher fat content. Integrate a lot of foods grown from the ground into your eating regimen. Fiber, vitamins, and minerals are abundant and naturally low in fat in these foods. Without putting additional strain on the digestive system, they supply essential nutrients. With little oil, vegetables can be eaten raw, steamed, roasted, or stir-fried. Fresh fruit can be eaten, blended into smoothies, or added to desserts and salads. Another essential component of a low-fat diet is whole grains. Settle on entire grains like earthy colored rice, quinoa, oats, and entire wheat items rather than refined grains. These have more nutrients and fiber, which help with digestion and keep energy levels consistent. Whole grains also help maintain a healthy microbiome in the gut, which is important for good digestion. Choose dairy products that are either fat-free or low-fat. Skim milk, low-fat yogurt, and diminished-fat cheddar can give the fundamental calcium and protein without the high-fat substance. On the off chance that lactose narrow-mindedness is an issue, without lactose choices, plant-based options like almond milk, soy milk, and coconut yogurt can be great substitutes. Cooking techniques play a critical part in keeping a low-fat eating routine. Instead of frying, you can use less oil by baking, grilling, steaming, or sautéing. Olive oil or avocado oil, two healthy cooking oils that contain beneficial fats but can still be difficult to digest in large quantities, should only be used in moderation. Additionally, cooking with non-stick pans and sprays can help cut down on the amount of oil needed to prepare food. By getting it and carrying out these low-fat eating routine fundamentals, you can more readily deal with your stomach-related wellbeing after gallbladder expulsion, limiting distress and advancing in general prosperity.

Foods to Avoid

After gallbladder expulsion, certain food varieties can intensify stomach-related distress and one ought to stay away from it to keep up with ideal stomach-related well-being. If you know which foods to avoid, you can make better decisions about your diet and avoid unpleasant symptoms like bloating, gas, and diarrhea. Foods with a lot of fat should be avoided at all costs. Full-fat dairy products, fatty meat cuts, fried foods, and processed snacks like chips and pastries are all examples of these. When bile is continuously flowing but in a less concentrated form, digesting foods high in fat requires more bile. Lessening the admission of these food varieties can help forestall over-burdening the stomach-related framework.

Additionally, you should avoid greasy foods, which frequently accompany high-fat foods. Oil and oils can be challenging to process and may prompt stomach-related trouble. This incorporates cheap food, weighty sauces, and varieties prepared in a lot of oil or spread. Picking better cooking techniques and diminishing the utilization of added fats can moderate these issues. Hot food sources can be aggravating to the stomach-related framework, particularly after gallbladder expulsion. Flavors like bean stew powder, hot sauce, and pepper can cause aggravation and lead to side effects like acid reflux or stomach torment. While certain individuals might endure gentle flavors, it's ideal to present them gradually and screen how your body answers. Although generally beneficial, high-fiber foods should be incorporated following surgery. If quickly consumed in large quantities, foods like beans, lentils, broccoli, and Brussels sprouts can cause gas and bloating. Your digestive system can adjust as you gradually increase your fiber intake, reducing discomfort. After the gallbladder surgery, some individuals may have issues with dairy products. Particularly, full-fat dairy products should be avoided. Plant-based or lactose-free alternatives may be beneficial if you suffer from lactose intolerance or difficulty digesting dairy products. Caffeine and liquor are different substances that can bother the stomach-related framework. Coffee, tea, and some sodas contain caffeine, which can cause diarrhea or discomfort by stimulating the digestive system. Liquor can likewise aggravate stomach fixing and impede absorption. Drinking these drinks less or avoiding them can help keep your digestive system healthy. Reduce consumption of processed foods, which frequently contain sugar, fat, and additives. These food varieties can be difficult to process and may add to stomach-related issues. Deciding on entire, natural food varieties can uphold better stomach-related well-being and prosperity. You can support a smoother transition to life without a gallbladder and reduce the risk of digestive discomfort by avoiding these problematic foods. Zeroing in on solid, effectively absorbable food sources will advance stomach-related capability and well-being.

Safe and Beneficial Foods

After gallbladder expulsion, certain food varieties can intensify stomach-related distress and one ought to stay away from it to keep up with ideal stomach-related well-being. If you know which foods to avoid, you can make better decisions about your diet and avoid unpleasant symptoms like bloating, gas, and diarrhea. Foods with a lot of fat should be avoided at all costs. Full-fat dairy products, fatty meat cuts, fried foods, and processed snacks like chips and pastries are all examples of these. When bile is continuously flowing but in a less concentrated form, digesting foods high in fat requires more bile. Lessening the admission of these food varieties can help forestall over-burdening the stomach-related framework.

Additionally, you should avoid greasy foods, which frequently accompany high-fat foods. Oil and oils can be challenging to process and may prompt stomach-related trouble. This incorporates cheap food, weighty sauces, and varieties prepared in a lot of oil or spread. Picking better cooking techniques and diminishing the utilization of added fats can moderate these issues. Hot food sources can be aggravating to the stomach-related framework, particularly after gallbladder expulsion. Flavors like bean stew powder, hot sauce, and pepper can cause aggravation and lead to side effects like acid reflux or stomach torment. While certain individuals might endure gentle flavors, it's ideal to present them gradually and screen how your body answers. Although generally beneficial, high-fiber foods should be incorporated following surgery. If quickly consumed in large quantities, foods like beans, lentils, broccoli, and Brussels sprouts can cause gas and bloating. Your digestive system can adjust as you gradually increase your fiber intake, reducing discomfort. After the gallbladder surgery, some individuals may have issues with dairy products. Particularly, full-fat dairy products should be avoided. Plant-based or lactose-free alternatives may be beneficial if you suffer from lactose intolerance or difficulty digesting dairy products. Caffeine and liquor are different substances that can bother the stomach-related framework. Coffee, tea, and some sodas contain caffeine, which can cause diarrhea or discomfort by stimulating the digestive system. Liquor can likewise aggravate stomach fixing and impede absorption. Drinking these drinks less or avoiding them can help keep your digestive system healthy. Reduce consumption of processed foods, which frequently contain sugar, fat, and additives. These food varieties can be difficult to process and may add to stomach-related issues. Deciding on entire, natural food varieties can uphold better stomach-related well-being and prosperity. You can support a smoother transition to life without a gallbladder and reduce the risk of digestive discomfort by avoiding these problematic foods. Zeroing in on solid, effectively absorbable food sources will advance stomach-related capability and well-being.

CHAPTER 3: STOCKING YOUR PANTRY

Must-Have Ingredients For Your Kitchen

It is essential to eat a low-fat diet to have the right ingredients in your kitchen. You will be able to prepare healthy meals without being tempted by unhealthy alternatives if your pantry, refrigerator, and freezer are well-equipped. Here is a broad manual for must-have fixings that help a fair, low-fat way of life.

WHOLE GRAINS

Brown Rice: A flexible and nutritious staple, brown rice is high in fiber and fundamental nutrients. Stir-fries, salads, and other side dishes can all be made with it as a base.

Quinoa: Quinoa is a great alternative to rice because it contains all nine essential amino acids and is known for its high protein content. It's fast to cook and functions admirably in servings of mixed greens, bowls, and as a side dish.

Oats: Oats are a great breakfast food because they are high in fiber and help keep you feeling energetic all day. Oatmeal, baking, and even savory dishes like meatloaf can all benefit from their use.

Whole Grain Pasta: Whole-grain pasta is a great alternative to regular pasta because it contains more nutrients and fiber. It goes well with a wide range of vegetables and sauces.

Whole Wheat Flour: Whole wheat flour is essential for baking and contains more nutrients and fiber than white flour. It can be used to make pancakes, muffins, bread, and other treats.

LEAN PROTEINS

Skinless Chicken Breasts: Chicken breasts are a staple of many low-fat diets because they are high in protein and can be prepared in a variety of ways, including baking and grilling.

Turkey: Both ground turkey and turkey bosoms are astounding low-fat protein sources. They are adaptable and can be used in casseroles as well as burgers.

Fish: Wealthy in omega-3 unsaturated fats, fish like salmon, mackerel, and cod are fundamental for a sound eating routine. Fatty fish should be included in moderation for better heart health.

Tofu and Tempeh: These are excellent flavors-absorbing plant-based proteins that are suitable for vegetarians and vegans. They can be barbecued, pan-seared, or added to soups and mixed greens.

Eggs and Egg Whites: Eggs are flexible and nutritious, while egg whites are a low-fat wellspring of protein. Bake, make omelets, and use them in frittatas.

LEGUMES

Black Beans: These are a nutritious addition to salads, soups, and casseroles because they contain a lot of protein and fiber.

Chickpeas: These are a great source of protein and fiber and can be used in salads, hummus, and other dishes.

Lentils: Lentils are great for soups, stews, and salads because they cook quickly and are full of nutrients. They are available in green, brown, and red varieties.

Kidney Beans: Kidney beans, another legume with a lot of protein, are great in chili, soups, and salads.

HEALTHY FATS

Olive Oil: This is ideal for salad dressings and cooking due to its high content of monounsaturated fats. It can be used sparingly to enhance flavors without introducing harmful fats.

Avocado Oil: Avocado oil—another healthy oil—provides heart-healthy fats and is ideal for high-heat cooking.

Nuts and Seeds: Nutritious and full of essential fatty acids, flaxseeds, chia seeds, and walnuts are all good choices. Snacks, salads, and smoothies are all good uses for them.

Nut Butters: Almond butter and peanut butter are good sources of healthy fats and protein. Choose varieties without added sugars or hydrogenated oils.

DAIRY AND DAIRY ALTERNATIVES

Low-Fat or Fat-Free Yogurt: High in protein and probiotics, yogurt is perfect for processing and can be utilized in breakfast bowls, smoothies, and as a base for dressings.

Skim Milk: It offers vitamin D and calcium without the fat of whole milk. It's great for cooking, cereal, and coffee.

Cheese: Select low-fat cheddar assortments to partake in the flavor without an abundance of fat. In moderation, cheese can be used in cooking, sandwiches, and salads.

Plant-Based Milks: Almond milk, soy milk, and oat milk are astounding dairy choices. They can be found in low-fat varieties and are frequently enriched with vitamins and minerals.

FRUITS AND VEGETABLES

Leafy Greens: Arugula, kale, and spinach are high in nutrients and low in calories. They can be utilized in plates of mixed greens, smoothies, and as a side dish.

Berries: Blueberries, strawberries, and raspberries are high in cancer-prevention agents and nutrients. They are ideally suited for nibbling, adding to grains, or making sweets.

Cruciferous Vegetables: Broccoli, cauliflower, and Brussels sprouts are plentiful in fiber and nutrients. They can be added to stir-fries, roasted, or steamed.

Root Vegetables: Beets, sweet potatoes, and carrots are all nutritious and adaptable. They can be simmered, pounded, or utilized in soups and stews.

Citrus Fruits: Oranges, lemons, and limes are high in L-ascorbic acid and add new flavors to dishes. They are suitable for use in beverages, marinades, and dressings.

PANTRY STAPLES

Canned Tomatoes: Indispensable for stews, soups, and sauces. Control your salt intake by choosing foods low in sodium.

Tomato Paste: Adds rich flavor to dishes and is helpful for thickening sauces.

Broth or Stock: When making soups, stews, and grains, low-sodium vegetable, chicken, or beef broth is essential.

Spices and Herbs: Spices like cumin, turmeric, and cinnamon, as well as fresh and dried herbs like basil, oregano, and thyme, should be kept on hand. These add flavor without fat.

Garlic and Onions: Essential for enhancing dishes' depth. They can be utilized in practically any appetizing recipe.

Vinegars: Dressings and marinades can benefit greatly from apple cider, red wine, and balsamic vinegar.

CONVENIENCE ITEMS

Frozen Vegetables: A fantastic alternative when fresh produce is unavailable. They are picked when they are at their most ripe, so most of their nutrients remain.

Frozen Fruits: Ideal for topping yogurt and cereal, smoothies, and desserts.

Whole Grain Bread and Tortillas: To get the most nutrients and fiber, make sure they are 100% whole grain.

Canned Beans: a simple and quick way to get protein and fiber. Rinse them to diminish sodium content.

Shopping Tips for a Low-Fat Diet

Taking on a low-fat eating routine includes something beyond removing high-fat food varieties; it requires smart preparation and vital shopping to guarantee you have nutritious, low-fat choices accessible. You can fill your pantry and refrigerator with ingredients that support your dietary goals and promote overall health by following these shopping tips.

Plan Your Meals and Make a List

Planning your meals is the first step toward effective shopping. Make a week-by-week feast plan that incorporates various low-fat, supplement-thick food varieties. Think about breakfast, lunch, supper, and tidbits. You can make a comprehensive shopping list that includes all of the ingredients you need by planning your meals. This will make it less tempting to buy unhealthy items on the spur of the moment. Keeping a detailed shopping list will help you stay focused and avoid forgetting important things. Sort your list by food groups like proteins, grains, dairy, fruits and vegetables, and pantry staples. This makes shopping more effective as well as guarantees you buy a fair scope of food varieties.

Focus on Fresh Produce

A low-fat diet should be based on fruits and vegetables. Naturally low in fat, these foods also contain many essential nutrients, fiber, and antioxidants. At each meal, try to include half of your plate with fruits and vegetables. While shopping, pick a wide assortment of brilliant produce to guarantee you get nutrients and minerals. Produce that is in season typically tastes better and is less expensive. Fresh, seasonal fruits and vegetables are seen at local farmers' markets. On the off chance that new produce isn't generally accessible, consider frozen choices, which hold the greater part of their supplements and can be similarly solid.

Choose Lean Proteins

Protein is a pivotal piece of any eating routine, however, picking low-fat sources is significant. While looking for meat, pick lean cuts like skinless chicken bosoms, turkey, and lean hamburger or pork cuts like flank or round. Before cooking, trim any visible fat. Fish is a great source of healthy fats and lean protein. Include a variety of fish in your diet, but focus on fish like salmon, mackerel, and sardines that are high in omega-3 fatty acids. In moderation, these fats can be easier to digest and are beneficial to heart health. For plant-based protein choices, stock up on beans, lentils, chickpeas, tofu, and tempeh. These are great for a low-fat diet because they are high in fiber and low in fat. Eggs, especially egg whites, are likewise a decent wellspring of low-fat protein.

Opt for Whole Grains

A diet low in fat cannot function without whole grains. They provide vitamins, minerals, and fiber, and help keep energy levels consistent. While looking for grains, pick brown rice, quinoa, bulgur, oats, and entire wheat items over their refined partners. To ensure that you are purchasing whole grain products, carefully read the labels. Search for terms like "100 percent entire grain" or "entire wheat" as the main fixing. Products with refined grains or enriched flour listed as the primary ingredient should be avoided.

Select Low-Fat Dairy

If you choose the right kinds, dairy products can be part of a low-fat diet. Pick low-fat or without-fat forms of milk, yogurt, and cheddar. These items give the important calcium and protein without the high-fat substance. Greek yogurt is especially beneficial due to its higher protein content and availability in low-fat varieties. For individuals who are lactose-prejudiced or inclined toward plant-based choices, there are numerous options accessible. Almond milk, soy milk, and coconut yogurt are great substitutes that are much of the time lower in fat than their dairy partners. Look for added sugars on the labels of plant-based dairy alternatives, and try to choose ones that are enriched with calcium and vitamin D.

Avoid Processed and High-Fat Foods

Processed foods frequently contain a lot of sodium, sugar, and unhealthy fats. Baked goods, ready-to-eat meals, packaged snacks, and fast food are all examples of these. Instead, concentrate on whole, unprocessed foods that are richer in nutrients. Avoid the aisles of chips, cookies, and other processed snacks when shopping. If you do need convenience foods, look for ones without added sugars or unhealthy fats and clean ingredient lists. Peruse names cautiously to comprehend what you're purchasing and stay away from items with hydrogenated oils or trans fats.

Check Labels for Hidden Fats

When shopping for a diet low in fat, it's important to read the labels. Indeed, even apparently solid items can contain stowed-away fats. Search for terms like "low-fat," "without fat," and "light" on the bundling, however, know that these can now and again be deceiving. Items marked as "low-fat" may contain added sugars to make up for the diminished fat, which can increment calorie content. Pay close attention to the serving sizes as well as the amount of cholesterol, trans fat, and saturated fat in each serving. The weight of the ingredients is listed first, so if fats or oils are near the top, the product may contain more fat than you think.

Shop the Perimeter

Most new and sound things are situated around the edge of the supermarket. Whole grains, dairy products, fruits and vegetables, and lean meats are all included in this. Shopping the border can assist you with keeping away from the inward passageways, which are many times loaded with handled and bundled food sources high in undesirable fats and sugars.

Be Mindful of Beverages

Drinks can be a secret wellspring of fats and sugars. Drink herbal teas, water, and other low-calorie, low-fat beverages. Energy drinks, sugary sodas, and high-fat drinks like milkshakes and full-fat lattes should be avoided. Plant-based milk alternatives and low-fat or fat-free milk are good options. Juices can be high in natural sugars, so choose 100% fruit juice with no added sugar and limit your consumption.

Buy in Bulk Wisely

Purchasing in mass can set aside cash and guarantee you generally have sound fixings close by. Nevertheless, it is essential to purchase things that you use frequently and have a long shelf life. Entire grains, vegetables, and nuts are superb contenders for mass buys. Make sure you have a strategy for using the perishable items you buy in bulk before they spoil. Freezing parts of new produce, meats, and arranged dinners can assist with broadening their timeframe of realistic usability and diminish squandering.

Embrace Healthy Fats

Not all fats are terrible. Healthy fats can be included in a low-fat diet in moderation because they are necessary for body function. These include healthy oils like olive oil and avocado oil, and fats from nuts, seeds, and avocados. These fats give fundamental unsaturated fats and can further develop heart wellbeing. When preparing meals and dressings, use these healthy fats sparingly. Use avocado as a spread instead of butter, for instance, or drizzle salads with a small amount of olive oil. In order to adhere to the recommended fat intake limits, portion control is essential.

Utilize Technology

Shopping for a low-fat diet can be made easier with the availability of numerous apps and online resources. You can use these tools to get nutrition facts, make shopping lists, and even get healthy recipe ideas based on what you already have. Utilizing a sustenance application can likewise assist you with following your fat admission and guarantee you are meeting your dietary objectives. You can also save money on healthy foods by downloading apps with digital coupons and deals from many grocery stores. By following these thorough shopping tips, you can settle on informed decisions that help a low-fat eating routine, guaranteeing you have the right fixings to get ready for nutritious feasts that advance stomach-related wellbeing and by and large prosperity.

Meal Prep Essentials

Preparing meals ahead of time is an essential part of eating well, especially for people who follow a low-fat diet. Viable feast prep can save time, decrease pressure, and guarantee you generally have nutritious dinners and tidbits close by. This comprehensive guide to the essentials of meal preparation will assist you in remaining organized and simplifying healthy eating.

Organize Your Kitchen

Meal preparation is based on a well-organized kitchen. Guarantee that your work area is spotless and deliberate to make cooking more charming and productive. Start by organizing your pantry, refrigerator, and freezer, decluttering your kitchen. Grains, canned goods, spices, and cooking oils are examples of similar items that belong together. Put resources into capacity arrangements like clear compartments and marks to keep everything noticeable and available. This not just assists you with seeing what you have initially yet in addition forestalls food squander. Orchestrate your kitchen devices and utensils such that they are simple to reach while cooking. Having a clean and efficient kitchen will make feast prep a smoother and more wonderful experience.

Essential Kitchen Tools

For effective meal preparation, having the right kitchen tools is essential. The following are essential items:

- **Sharp Knives:** For chopping vegetables, slicing meat, and more, you need a set of good, sharp knives.

- **Cutting Boards:** Cross-contamination is prevented by using multiple cutting boards. Consider having separate sheets for meats, vegetables, and bread.

- **Measuring Cups and Spoons:** Exact estimation is vital for following recipes and part control.

- **Mixing Bowls:** Mixing ingredients, marinating meats, and making salads all require a variety of sizes.

- **Non-Stick Pans and Pots:**These are perfect for low-oil cooking.

- **Baking Sheets and Pans:** Useful for baking fish, roasting vegetables, and making low-fat desserts.

- **Blender or Food Processor:** essential for quickly chopping ingredients and making smoothies, soups, and sauces.

- **Storage Containers:** Purchase a variety of airtight containers for storing cooked meals and prepared ingredients. Glass containers are a great choice because they are safe for use in the microwave and do not retain stains or odors.

- **Slow Cooker or Instant Pot:** With minimal effort, these appliances are ideal for batch-cooking grains, stews, and soups.

- **Spiralizer:** A useful tool for making vegetable noodles, which are an alternative to pasta that is low in fat and carbs.

- **Batch Cooking and Freezing:** Cluster cooking is the foundation of dinner prep. It involves making a lot of staple foods in large quantities that can be used throughout the week. This not only saves you time but also guarantees that you will always have healthy options available to you. How to effectively cook meals in batches and freeze them.

- **Choose Recipes Wisely:** Choose recipes that are versatile and good for freezing. Grain-based dishes, stews, casseroles, and soups are excellent choices.

- **Cook in Bulk:** Get ready for enormous groups of grains like brown rice, quinoa, and whole-grain pasta. Cook lean proteins like chicken bosoms, turkey, and fish. Various vegetables can be roasted.

- **Portion Control:** Get ready for enormous groups of grains like brown rice, quinoa, and whole-grain pasta. Cook lean proteins like chicken bosoms, turkey, and fish. Various vegetables can be roasted.

- **Label and Date:** Name and date all holders before putting them in the cooler. This ensures that you use older items first and helps you keep track of what you have.

- **Prepping Vegetables and Fruits:**During the week, preparing fruits and vegetables ahead of time saves time and encourages healthier eating. To begin, follow these steps:

- **Wash and Dry:** Wash all produce thoroughly to remove dirt and pesticides. To dry greens, spin them in a salad spinner.

- **Chop and Slice:** Slice vegetables into small pieces. Refrigerate them in airtight containers or zip-lock bags. A few vegetables, similar to carrots and celery, can be put away in water to keep them fresh.

- **Fruit Prep:** Cut natural products like berries, melons, and apples and store them in holders. A squeeze of lemon juice can help preserve the color of fruits that brown quickly, like apples.

- **Use Ready-to-Eat Snacks:** Pre-segment snacks, for example, carrot sticks, ringer pepper cuts, and berries into individual servings. This makes it simple to get a sound nibble in a hurry.

Cooking Methods

Picking health cooking techniques is fundamental for keeping a low-fat eating routine. Here are a few methods to consider:

- **Grilling:** Flavor can be added without using too much oil by grilling. Utilize a barbecue skillet or outside barbecue for meats, vegetables, and even fruits.
- **Baking and Roasting:** A wide range of foods, from vegetables to lean proteins, can be baked or roasted with little oil.
- **Steaming:** Steaming jam supplements and flavor in vegetables and fish. Utilize a liner bushel or an electric liner.
- **Sautéing:** Use a non-stick dish and cooking splashes to sauté vegetables and lean proteins with negligible oil.
- **Slow Cooking:** Slow cookers are ideal for quickly and easily making large batches of soups, stews, and casseroles. Simply add fixings and let it cook for more than a few hours.

- **Blending:** Smoothies, soups, and sauces that are nutritious and easy to digest can all be made with the help of a blender.

Plan for Variety and Balance

A well-balanced diet is guaranteed when you plan meals that include a variety of food groups. Aim to include:

- **Lean Proteins:** Eggs, tofu, fish, chicken, turkey, and legumes.
- **Whole Grains:** Oats, whole grain pasta, quinoa, and brown rice.
- **Fruits and Vegetables:** A wide range of colors and types to guarantee a diverse supply of nutrients.
- **Healthy Fats:** Healthy oils, avocado, nuts, and seeds, in moderation.
- **Dairy or Dairy Alternatives:** ogurt with low fat, skim milk, or plant-based milks with added nutrients.

Healthy Snacks

Preparing healthy snacks can keep you from going after undesirable choices. Here are a few concepts:

- **Nuts and Seeds:** Divide the nuts and seeds into small bags or containers beforehand. They give protein and solid fats.
- **Fruit and Yogurt:** For a quick and healthy snack, mix low-fat yogurt with fresh fruit.
- **Vegetable Sticks and Hummus:** Hummus-topped carrot sticks, cucumber slices, and bell pepper strips are excellent low-fat snacks.
- **Whole Grain Crackers:** Match with low-fat cheddar or nut margarine for a delightful bite.

Storage and Organization

Appropriate capacity is vital for keeping prepared dinners new. Here are a few hints:

- **Airtight Containers:** To keep food fresh for longer, use containers that seal tightly.

- **Clear Containers:** Clear compartments permit you to see what's inside without opening them, assisting with monitoring your prepared food.
- **Stackable Containers:** These conserve freezer and refrigerator space.
- **Freezer Bags:** Soups, stews, and sauces can be stored in freezer bags. To freeze, lay them flat, and then stack them to save space.
- **Vacuum Sealers:** Foods can be preserved for longer by vacuum sealers by removing air before sealing.

Scheduling Meal Prep

It is essential to set aside specific time for meal preparation. Pick a little while every week to zero in on preparing feasts. Many individuals find that Sunday functions admirably as it sets them up for the impending week. Give yourself a few hours to shop, prepare, cook, and store food. By integrating these feast prep basics into your daily practice, you can guarantee that you generally have sound, low-fat dinners all set. This supports your dietary objectives as well as recovery time and diminishes pressure, making smart dieting more manageable   and   agreeable.

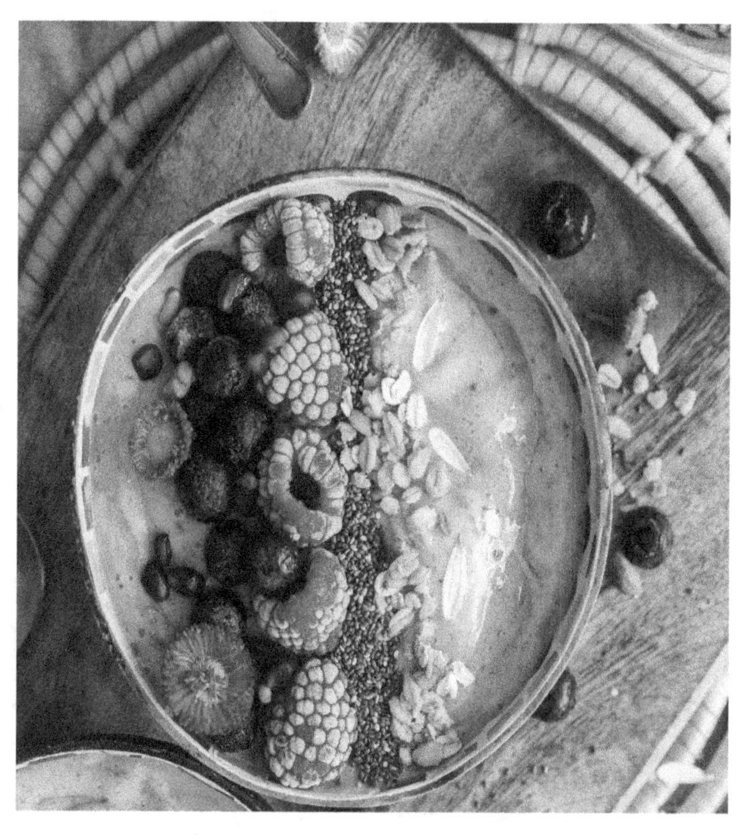

CHAPTER 4: BREAKFAST RECIPES

ENERGIZING MORNING MEALS

Breakfast Quinoa with Apples and Cinnamon

A wholesome and nutritious option. Rich in fiber and provides a warm, comforting start to the day.

Prep Time: 10 minutes
Cooking Time: 15 minutes
Serving Size: 1 cup (serves 2)

Ingredients: • 1/2 cup quinoa • 1 cup water • 1/2 cup diced apples • 1/4 teaspoon ground cinnamon • 1/2 cup low-fat milk • 2 tablespoons chopped walnuts • 2 teaspoons honey (optional)

Instructions:

1. Rinse quinoa under cold water. In a saucepan, bring 1 cup of water to a boil. Add quinoa, reduce

heat to low, cover, and simmer for about 15 minutes, or until water is absorbed and quinoa is tender.

2. In a bowl, combine cooked quinoa, diced apples, and ground cinnamon.

3. Heat low-fat milk in a microwave or stovetop until warm.

4. Pour warm milk over the quinoa mixture.

5. Top with chopped walnuts and drizzle with honey if desired.

Nutritional Information (per cup): • Calories: 250 • Protein: 6g • Carbohydrates: 47g • Dietary Fiber: 6g • Fat: 6g • Saturated Fat: 1g • Sodium: 60mg • Potassium: 270mg • Phosphorus: 150mg

Spinach and Tomato Egg White Scramble

A light and protein-packed breakfast that's quick to prepare and gentle on your digestive system.

Prep Time: 5 minutes

Cooking Time: 10 minutes

Serving Size: 1 cup (serves 2)

Ingredients: • 4 large egg whites • 1 cup fresh spinach, chopped • 1/2 cup cherry tomatoes, halved • 1/4 teaspoon garlic powder • Salt and pepper to taste • 1 teaspoon olive oil

Instructions:

1. In a bowl, whisk egg whites with garlic powder, salt, and pepper.
2. Heat olive oil in a non-stick skillet over medium heat. Add spinach and tomatoes, and cook until spinach is wilted.
3. Pour egg whites into the skillet and cook, stirring gently, until eggs are fully cooked and scrambled.

Nutritional Information (per cup): • Calories: 80 • Protein: 14g • Carbohydrates: 3g • Dietary Fiber: 1g • Fat: 2g • Saturated Fat: 0.5g • Sodium: 180mg • Potassium: 400mg • Phosphorus: 200mg

Oatmeal with Berries and Flaxseeds

A high-fiber, antioxidant-rich breakfast that's perfect for sustaining energy levels throughout the morning.

Prep Time: 5 minutes

Cooking Time: 10 minutes

Serving Size: 1 cup (serves 2)

Ingredients: • 1 cup rolled oats • 2 cups water • 1/2 cup mixed berries (blueberries, strawberries, raspberries) • 1 tablespoon ground flaxseeds • 1 teaspoon honey (optional) • 1/4 cup low-fat milk

Instructions:

1. In a saucepan, bring water to a boil. Add rolled oats and reduce heat to low. Simmer for about 10 minutes, stirring occasionally, until oats are cooked.
2. Stir in mixed berries and ground flaxseeds.
3. Divide oatmeal into bowls, drizzle with honey if desired, and pour a little milk over each serving.

Nutritional Information (per cup): • Calories: 220 • Protein: 6g • Carbohydrates: 39g • Dietary Fiber: 8g • Fat: 4g • Saturated Fat: 0.5g • Sodium: 10mg • Potassium: 250mg • Phosphorus: 180mg

Greek Yogurt Parfait with Honey and Almonds

A creamy and crunchy breakfast that's high in protein and healthy fats.

Prep Time: 5 minutes
Serving Size: 1 cup (serves 2)

Ingredients: • 1 cup plain Greek yogurt • 1/4 cup granola (low-fat) • 1/4 cup sliced almonds • 1 tablespoon honey • 1/2 cup mixed berries (blueberries, raspberries)

Instructions:

1. In a glass or bowl, layer half of the Greek yogurt.
2. Add a layer of mixed berries and granola.
3. Top with the remaining Greek yogurt.
4. Sprinkle with sliced almonds and drizzle with honey.

Nutritional Information (per cup): • Calories: 300 • Protein: 15g • Carbohydrates: 40g • Dietary Fiber: 5g • Fat: 10g • Saturated Fat: 1.5g • Sodium: 80mg • Potassium: 300mg • Phosphorus: 250mg

Avocado Toast with Poached Eggs

A nutrient-dense breakfast that combines healthy fats and protein to keep you full and energized.

Prep Time: 5 minutes
Cooking Time: 10 minutes
Serving Size: 1 slice (serves 2)

Ingredients: • 2 slices whole-grain bread • 1 ripe avocado • 2 large eggs • 1 teaspoon lemon juice • Salt and pepper to taste • 1/4 teaspoon red pepper flakes (optional)

Instructions:

1. Toast the whole-grain bread slices.
2. In a small bowl, mash the avocado with lemon juice, salt, and pepper.
3. Spread the avocado mixture on the toasted bread.
4. Poach the eggs by bringing a pot of water to a simmer. Crack each egg into a small bowl and gently slide into the water. Cook for about 3-4

minutes, until whites are set but yolks are still runny.

5. Place a poached egg on each avocado toast and sprinkle with red pepper flakes if desired.

Nutritional Information (per slice): • Calories: 300 • Protein: 12g • Carbohydrates: 28g • Dietary Fiber: 8g • Fat: 18g • Saturated Fat: 3g • Sodium: 250mg • Potassium: 600mg • Phosphorus: 200mg

Smoothie Bowl with Spinach and Banana

A refreshing and nutrient-packed breakfast that's easy to digest and full of vitamins.

Prep Time: 10 minutes
Serving Size: 1 bowl (serves 2)

Ingredients: • 1 banana • 1 cup fresh spinach • 1/2 cup frozen mixed berries • 1/2 cup unsweetened almond milk • 1 tablespoon chia seeds • 1 tablespoon almond butter • 1/4 cup granola (low-fat)

Instructions:

1. In a blender, combine banana, spinach, frozen berries, and almond milk. Blend until smooth.
2. Pour smoothie into bowls.
3. Top with chia seeds, almond butter, and granola.

Nutritional Information (per bowl): • Calories: 280 • Protein: 7g • Carbohydrates: 45g • Dietary Fiber: 9g • Fat: 10g • Saturated Fat: 1g • Sodium: 150mg • Potassium: 700mg • Phosphorus: 150mg

Cottage Cheese with Pineapple and Chia Seeds

A protein-rich breakfast with a touch of sweetness and a boost of omega-3s.

Prep Time: 5 minutes

Serving Size: 1 cup (serves 2)

Ingredients: • 1 cup low-fat cottage cheese • 1/2 cup pineapple chunks (fresh or canned in juice) • 2 teaspoons chia seeds • 1 teaspoon honey (optional)

Instructions:

1. In a bowl, mix cottage cheese with pineapple chunks.
2. Sprinkle chia seeds on top.
3. Drizzle with honey if desired.

Nutritional Information (per cup): • Calories: 200 • Protein: 18g • Carbohydrates: 20g • Dietary Fiber: 3g • Fat: 5g • Saturated Fat: 2g • Sodium: 400mg • Potassium: 350mg • Phosphorus: 250mg

Whole Grain Pancakes with Blueberries

A delicious and filling breakfast that combines whole grains with the antioxidant power of blueberries.

Prep Time: 10 minutes
Cooking Time: 15 minutes
Serving Size: 2 pancakes (serves 2)

Ingredients: • 1/2 cup whole wheat flour • 1/2 teaspoon baking powder • 1/4 teaspoon baking soda • 1/4 teaspoon salt • 1/2 cup low-fat buttermilk • 1 egg white • 1 tablespoon honey • 1/2 cup fresh blueberries

Instructions:

1. In a bowl, mix whole wheat flour, baking powder, baking soda, and salt.
2. In another bowl, whisk together buttermilk, egg white, and honey. Add to the dry ingredients and stir until just combined.
3. Gently fold in blueberries.
4. Heat a non-stick skillet over medium heat and lightly coat with cooking spray. Pour batter onto skillet to form pancakes.
5. Cook until bubbles form on the surface and edges look set, then flip and cook until golden brown.

Nutritional Information (per 2 pancakes): • Calories: 220 • Protein: 8g • Carbohydrates: 40g • Dietary Fiber: 6g • Fat: 3g • Saturated Fat: 1g • Sodium: 300mg • Potassium: 200mg • Phosphorus: 180mg

Apple Cinnamon Overnight Oats

A convenient and hearty breakfast that's ready to go in the morning, packed with fiber and flavor.

Prep Time: 10 minutes

Refrigeration Time: Overnight

Serving Size: 1 cup (serves 2)

Ingredients: • 1 cup rolled oats • 1 cup low-fat milk or almond milk • 1/2 cup unsweetened applesauce • 1/2 teaspoon ground cinnamon • 1 tablespoon chia seeds • 1 teaspoon honey (optional)

Instructions:

1. In a bowl or jar, mix rolled oats, milk, applesauce, ground cinnamon, and chia seeds.
2. Stir well to combine and cover.
3. Refrigerate overnight.
4. In the morning, stir the oats and add honey if desired before serving.

Nutritional Information (per cup): • Calories: 250 • Protein: 8g • Carbohydrates: 45g • Dietary Fiber: 8g • Fat: 5g • Saturated Fat: 1g • Sodium: 50mg • Potassium: 300mg • Phosphorus: 200mg

Veggie Breakfast Burrito

A savory and filling breakfast that's easy to make and full of vegetables and lean protein.

Prep Time: 10 minutes

Cooking Time: 10 minutes

Serving Size: 1 burrito (serves 2)

Ingredients: • 4 egg whites • 1/2 cup black beans, drained and rinsed • 1/2 cup diced bell peppers • 1/4 cup diced onions • 1/4 cup diced tomatoes • 1/2 teaspoon ground cumin • Salt and pepper to taste • 2 whole wheat tortillas • 1/4 cup salsa • 1/4 cup low-fat shredded cheese (optional)

Instructions:

1. In a non-stick skillet, cook bell peppers, onions, and tomatoes over medium heat until softened.
2. Add black beans, ground cumin, salt, and pepper, and cook until heated through.
3. In another skillet, scramble egg whites until cooked.

4. Warm whole wheat tortillas in a microwave or on a skillet.

5. Assemble burritos by placing scrambled eggs, vegetable mixture, salsa, and shredded cheese (if using) in the center of each tortilla. Roll up and serve.

Nutritional Information (per burrito): • Calories: 300 • Protein: 20g • Carbohydrates: 40g • Dietary Fiber: 10g • Fat: 5g • Saturated Fat: 1g • Sodium: 600mg • Potassium: 600mg • Phosphorus: 250mg

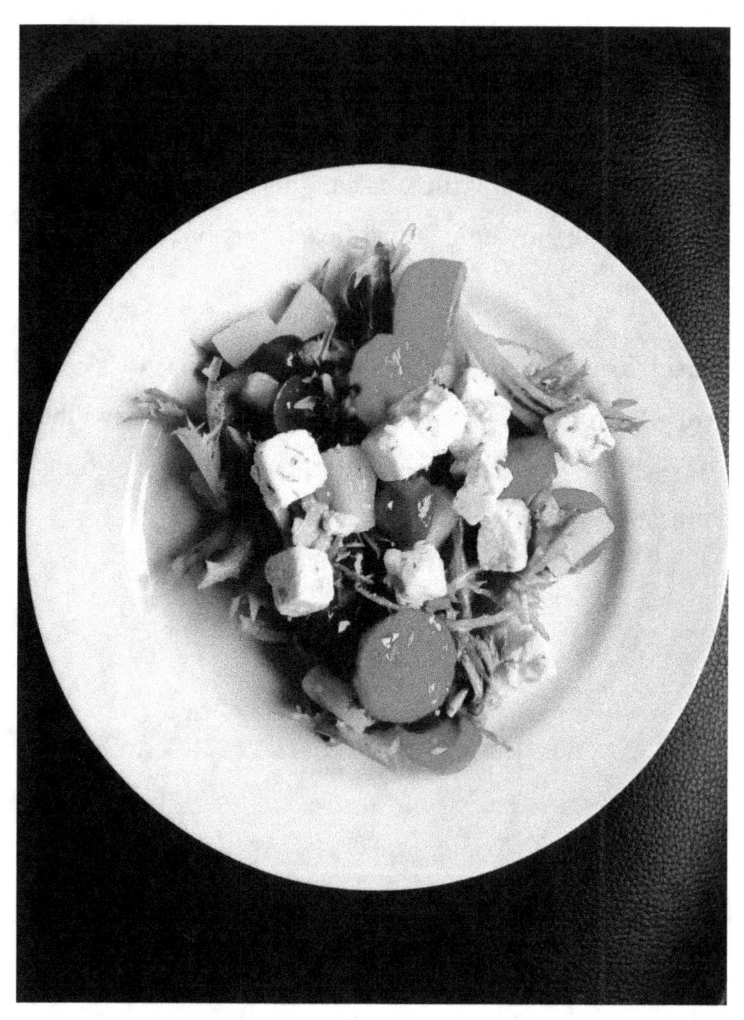

CHAPTER 5: LUNCH RECIPES

QUICK AND EASY LUNCHES

Grilled Chicken and Avocado Wrap

A light and flavorful wrap that's high in protein and healthy fats, perfect for a quick lunch.

Prep Time: 10 minutes

Cooking Time: 10 minutes

Serving Size: 1 wrap (serves 2)

Ingredients: • 2 small boneless, skinless chicken breasts • 1 avocado, sliced • 1 cup mixed greens • 1/2 cup cherry tomatoes, halved • 2 whole wheat tortillas • 1 tablespoon olive oil • 1 teaspoon lemon juice • Salt and pepper to taste

Instructions: Season the chicken breasts with salt and pepper. Heat olive oil in a non-stick skillet over medium heat. Grill the chicken breasts for about 5 minutes on each side, or until fully cooked. Slice the chicken into strips. In a small bowl, toss the avocado slices with lemon juice to prevent browning. Lay the tortillas flat and fill each with mixed greens, cherry tomatoes, grilled chicken, and avocado slices. Roll up the tortillas and serve immediately.

Nutritional Information (per wrap): • Calories: 350 • Protein: 30g • Carbohydrates: 30g • Dietary Fiber: 10g • Fat: 15g • Saturated Fat: 2g • Sodium: 400mg • Potassium: 800mg • Phosphorus: 250mg

Mediterranean Chickpea Salad

A refreshing and filling salad with a Mediterranean flair, packed with fiber and plant-based protein.

Prep Time: 15 minutes
Serving Size: 2 cups (serves 2)

Ingredients: • 1 can chickpeas, drained and rinsed • 1 cup cherry tomatoes, halved • 1/2 cucumber, diced • 1/4 red onion, finely chopped • 1/4 cup feta cheese, crumbled • 2 tablespoons olive oil • 1 tablespoon red wine vinegar • 1 teaspoon dried oregano • Salt and pepper to taste

Instructions: In a large bowl, combine chickpeas, cherry tomatoes, cucumber, red onion, and feta cheese. In a small bowl, whisk together olive oil, red wine vinegar, oregano, salt, and pepper. Pour the dressing over the salad and toss to combine. Serve immediately or refrigerate for up to one day.

Nutritional Information (per cup): • Calories: 250 • Protein: 10g • Carbohydrates: 30g • Dietary Fiber: 8g • Fat: 10g • Saturated Fat: 2g • Sodium: 400mg • Potassium: 300mg • Phosphorus: 200mg

Quinoa and Black Bean Salad

A nutritious and satisfying salad that combines quinoa and black beans with fresh vegetables.

Prep Time: 10 minutes
Cooking Time: 15 minutes
Serving Size: 2 cups (serves 2)

Ingredients: • 1/2 cup quinoa • 1 cup water • 1 can black beans, drained and rinsed • 1/2 red bell pepper, diced • 1/2 yellow bell pepper, diced • 1/4 cup chopped cilantro • 2 tablespoons lime juice • 1 tablespoon olive oil • Salt and pepper to taste

Instructions: Rinse quinoa under cold water. In a saucepan, bring 1 cup of water to a boil. Add quinoa, reduce heat to low, cover, and simmer for about 15 minutes, or until water is absorbed and quinoa is tender. In a large bowl, combine cooked quinoa, black beans, bell peppers, and cilantro. In a small bowl, whisk together lime juice, olive oil, salt, and pepper. Pour the dressing over the salad and toss to combine. Serve immediately or refrigerate for up to two days.

Nutritional Information (per cup): • Calories: 260 • Protein: 9g • Carbohydrates: 45g • Dietary Fiber: 10g • Fat: 6g • Saturated Fat: 1g • Sodium: 200mg • Potassium: 500mg • Phosphorus: 250mg

Turkey and Hummus Pita

A quick and healthy pita sandwich that's perfect for a light lunch, with lean protein and creamy hummus.

Prep Time: 10 minutes

Serving Size: 1 pita (serves 2)

Ingredients: • 2 whole wheat pitas • 4 ounces sliced turkey breast • 1/2 cup hummus • 1 cup mixed greens • 1/2 cucumber, sliced • 1/4 cup shredded carrots

Instructions: Cut each pita in half to create pockets. Spread hummus inside each pita half. Fill each pita with sliced turkey, mixed greens, cucumber, and shredded carrots. Serve immediately.

Nutritional Information (per pita): • Calories: 300 • Protein: 18g • Carbohydrates: 40g • Dietary Fiber: 8g • Fat: 8g • Saturated Fat: 1g • Sodium: 600mg • Potassium: 400mg • Phosphorus: 200mg

Lentil and Veggie Soup

A hearty and nourishing soup that's easy to prepare and packed with vegetables and lentils.

Prep Time: 10 minutes
Cooking Time: 30 minutes
Serving Size: 2 cups (serves 2)

Ingredients: • 1/2 cup dried lentils • 4 cups vegetable broth • 1 carrot, diced • 1 celery stalk, diced • 1/2 onion, diced • 1 clove garlic, minced • 1 can diced tomatoes • 1

teaspoon dried thyme • 1 bay leaf • Salt and pepper to taste

Instructions: In a large pot, combine lentils, vegetable broth, carrot, celery, onion, garlic, diced tomatoes, thyme, and bay leaf. Bring to a boil, then reduce heat and simmer for about 30 minutes, or until lentils and vegetables are tender. Remove bay leaf, season with salt and pepper, and serve.

Nutritional Information (per cup): • Calories: 180 • Protein: 10g • Carbohydrates: 30g • Dietary Fiber: 10g • Fat: 1g • Saturated Fat: 0g • Sodium: 500mg • Potassium: 400mg • Phosphorus: 150mg

Tuna Salad Lettuce Wraps

A light and crunchy lunch option that's low in fat and high in protein.

Prep Time: 10 minutes
Serving Size: 2 wraps (serves 2)

Ingredients: • 1 can tuna in water, drained • 2 tablespoons plain Greek yogurt • 1 tablespoon lemon juice • 1 celery stalk, diced • 1/4 red onion, finely chopped • Salt and pepper to taste • 4 large lettuce leaves

Instructions: In a bowl, mix tuna, Greek yogurt, lemon juice, celery, red onion, salt, and pepper until well combined. Spoon the tuna mixture onto the center of each lettuce leaf. Roll up the lettuce leaves to create wraps and serve.

Nutritional Information (per wrap): • Calories: 150 • Protein: 20g • Carbohydrates: 5g • Dietary Fiber: 2g • Fat: 3g • Saturated Fat: 0.5g • Sodium: 300mg • Potassium: 200mg • Phosphorus: 150mg

Cucumber and Avocado Sushi Rolls

A refreshing and light lunch option that's fun to make and perfect for a healthy meal.

Prep Time: 15 minutes
Cooking Time: 20 minutes
Serving Size: 6 rolls (serves 2)

Ingredients: • 1/2 cup sushi rice • 1 cup water • 2 sheets nori (seaweed) • 1/2 cucumber, sliced into thin strips • 1 avocado, sliced • 1 tablespoon rice vinegar • 1 teaspoon sugar • 1/4 teaspoon salt

Instructions: Rinse sushi rice under cold water. In a saucepan, combine rice and water, bring to a boil, reduce heat, cover, and simmer for 20 minutes, or until water is absorbed and rice is tender. In a small bowl, mix rice vinegar, sugar, and salt. Stir into the cooked rice and let cool slightly. Lay nori sheets flat and spread a thin layer of rice over each, leaving a 1-inch border at the top. Arrange cucumber and avocado slices over the rice. Roll up the nori tightly, using a little water to seal the edges. Cut into 6 pieces each and serve.

Nutritional Information (per roll): • Calories: 200 • Protein: 4g • Carbohydrates: 36g • Dietary Fiber: 4g • Fat: 6g • Saturated Fat: 1g • Sodium: 150mg • Potassium: 300mg • Phosphorus: 100mg

Chicken and Vegetable Stir-Fry

A quick and easy stir-fry that's full of lean protein and fresh vegetables.

Prep Time: 10 minutes

Cooking Time: 10 minutes

Serving Size: 2 cups (serves 2)

Ingredients: • 2 small boneless, skinless chicken breasts, sliced • 1 cup broccoli florets • 1 red bell pepper, sliced • 1 carrot, sliced • 1 clove garlic, minced • 1 tablespoon soy sauce • 1 tablespoon olive oil • 1/2 teaspoon ginger, grated

Instructions: Heat olive oil in a large skillet over medium-high heat. Add chicken slices and cook until browned and cooked through. Add broccoli, bell pepper, carrot, and garlic to the skillet. Cook for about 5 minutes, or until vegetables are tender. Stir in soy sauce and grated ginger. Cook for an additional 2 minutes, then serve.

Nutritional Information (per cup): • Calories: 250 • Protein: 25g • Carbohydrates: 15g • Dietary Fiber: 5g • Fat: 10g • Saturated Fat: 2g • Sodium: 400mg • Potassium: 600mg • Phosphorus: 200mg

Egg and Spinach Salad

A simple and nutritious salad that's quick to prepare and full of vitamins and protein.

Prep Time: 10 minutes
Serving Size: 2 cups (serves 2)

Ingredients: • 4 hard-boiled eggs, sliced • 4 cups baby spinach • 1/2 cup cherry tomatoes, halved • 1/4 red onion, thinly sliced • 1 tablespoon olive oil • 1 tablespoon balsamic vinegar • Salt and pepper to taste

Instructions: In a large bowl, combine baby spinach, cherry tomatoes, and red onion. Top with sliced hard-boiled eggs. In a small bowl, whisk together olive oil, balsamic vinegar, salt, and pepper. Drizzle the dressing over the salad and toss to combine. Serve immediately.

Nutritional Information (per cup): • Calories: 180 • Protein: 10g • Carbohydrates: 5g • Dietary Fiber: 2g • Fat: 14g • Saturated Fat: 3g • Sodium: 150mg • Potassium: 500mg • Phosphorus: 150mg

Sweet Potato and Black Bean Tacos

A tasty and filling taco recipe that's perfect for a quick and healthy lunch.

Prep Time: 10 minutes
Cooking Time: 20 minutes
Serving Size: 2 tacos (serves 2)

Ingredients: • 1 large sweet potato, peeled and diced • 1 can black beans, drained and rinsed • 1 teaspoon ground cumin • 1/2 teaspoon chili powder • 1 tablespoon olive oil • Salt and pepper to taste • 4 small corn tortillas • 1/4 cup salsa • 1/4 cup chopped cilantro

Instructions: Preheat oven to 400°F (200°C). Toss diced sweet potato with olive oil, ground cumin, chili powder, salt, and pepper. Spread on a baking sheet and roast for about 20 minutes, or until tender. In a small saucepan, heat black beans until warm. Warm corn tortillas in a microwave or on a skillet. Assemble tacos by filling each tortilla with roasted sweet potato, black beans, salsa, and chopped cilantro. Serve immediately.

Nutritional Information (per taco): • Calories: 200 • Protein: 6g • Carbohydrates: 36g • Dietary Fiber: 8g • Fat: 5g • Saturated Fat: 1g • Sodium: 300mg • Potassium: 400mg • Phosphorus: 150mg

Zucchini Noodles with Pesto

A light and refreshing dish that's low in carbs and full of flavor.

Prep Time: 10 minutes
Cooking Time: 10 minutes
Serving Size: 2 cups (serves 2)

Ingredients: • 2 medium zucchinis, spiralized • 1/4 cup basil pesto • 1/4 cup cherry tomatoes, halved • 2 tablespoons grated Parmesan cheese (optional) • Salt and pepper to taste

Instructions: Heat a non-stick skillet over medium heat. Add spiralized zucchini and cook for about 3-4 minutes, or until slightly tender. Remove from heat and toss with basil pesto. Add cherry tomatoes and sprinkle with grated Parmesan cheese if desired. Season with salt and pepper and serve immediately.

Nutritional Information (per cup): • Calories: 150 • Protein: 4g • Carbohydrates: 10g • Dietary Fiber: 4g • Fat: 10g • Saturated Fat: 2g • Sodium: 200mg • Potassium: 400mg • Phosphorus: 100mg

BONUS HERE:

Scan the QR code

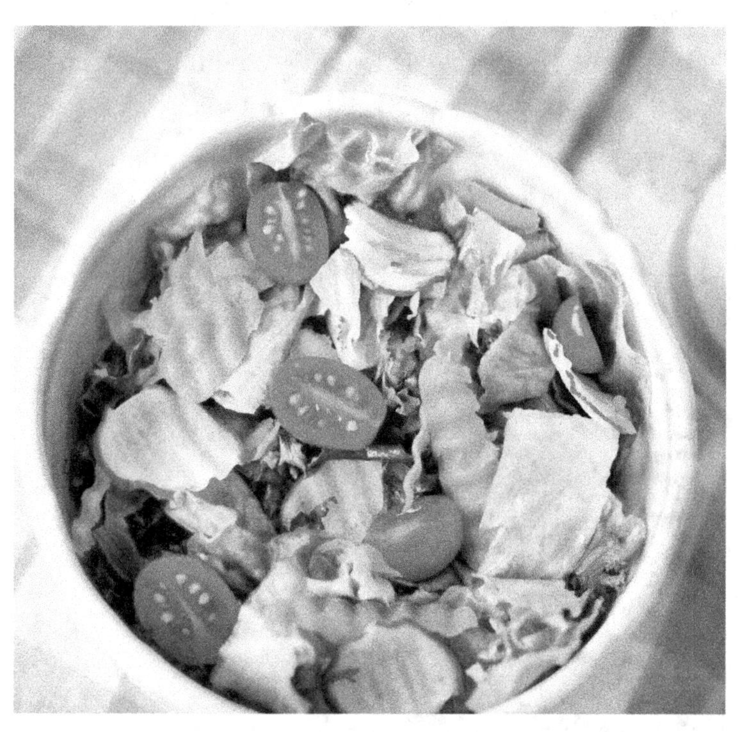

CHAPTER 6: DINNER RECIPES

Satisfying Main Courses

Lemon Herb Baked Chicken

A simple and flavorful chicken dish that is light and easy to prepare. Perfect for a healthy dinner.

Prep Time: 10 minutes
Cooking Time: 25 minutes
Serving Size: 1 chicken breast (serves 2)

Ingredients: • 2 boneless, skinless chicken breasts • 2 tablespoons olive oil • Juice of 1 lemon • 2 cloves garlic, minced • 1 teaspoon dried thyme • 1 teaspoon dried rosemary • Salt and pepper to taste

Instructions: Preheat the oven to 375°F (190°C). In a small bowl, whisk together olive oil, lemon juice, garlic, thyme, rosemary, salt, and pepper. Place the chicken breasts in a baking dish and pour the lemon herb mixture over them, ensuring they are well-coated. Bake for 25 minutes, or until the chicken is cooked through and no longer pink in the center. Serve immediately.

Nutritional Information (per chicken breast): • Calories: 300 • Protein: 30g • Carbohydrates: 2g • Dietary Fiber: 0g • Fat: 18g • Saturated Fat: 3g • Sodium: 200mg • Potassium: 500mg • Phosphorus: 250mg

Spaghetti with Tomato Basil Sauce

A classic pasta dish that's light and packed with flavor. Ideal for a quick and easy dinner.

Prep Time: 10 minutes
Cooking Time: 15 minutes
Serving Size: 1 cup (serves 2)

Ingredients: • 4 ounces whole wheat spaghetti • 2 cups cherry tomatoes, halved • 2 cloves garlic, minced • 1 tablespoon olive oil • 1/4 cup fresh basil, chopped • Salt and pepper to taste • 1/4 cup grated Parmesan cheese (optional)

Instructions: Cook the spaghetti according to package instructions. In a large skillet, heat olive oil over medium heat. Add garlic and cherry tomatoes, cooking until tomatoes are softened and garlic is fragrant. Add cooked spaghetti to the skillet and toss to combine. Stir in fresh basil and season with salt and pepper. Sprinkle with Parmesan cheese if desired and serve immediately.

Nutritional Information (per cup): • Calories: 320 • Protein: 10g • Carbohydrates: 56g • Dietary Fiber: 10g • Fat: 9g • Saturated Fat: 2g • Sodium: 150mg • Potassium: 600mg • Phosphorus: 200mg

Grilled Salmon with Asparagus

A healthy and delicious dish that combines the rich flavor of salmon with tender asparagus.

Prep Time: 10 minutes
Cooking Time: 15 minutes
Serving Size: 1 salmon fillet (serves 2)

Ingredients: • 2 salmon fillets • 1 bunch asparagus, trimmed • 2 tablespoons olive oil • Juice of 1 lemon • 1 teaspoon dried dill • Salt and pepper to taste

Instructions: Preheat the grill to medium-high heat. In a small bowl, whisk together olive oil, lemon juice, dill, salt, and pepper. Brush the salmon fillets and asparagus with the olive oil mixture. Grill the salmon for about 6-8 minutes on each side, or until the fish flakes easily with a fork. Grill the asparagus for about 5 minutes, turning occasionally, until tender. Serve immediately.

Nutritional Information (per salmon fillet): • Calories: 350 • Protein: 30g • Carbohydrates: 7g • Dietary Fiber: 4g • Fat: 22g • Saturated Fat: 3g • Sodium: 200mg • Potassium: 800mg • Phosphorus: 300mg

Quinoa Stuffed Bell Peppers

A colorful and nutritious dish that's both satisfying and easy to make.

Prep Time: 15 minutes
Cooking Time: 30 minutes
Serving Size: 1 pepper (serves 2)

Ingredients: • 2 large bell peppers, halved and seeded • 1/2 cup quinoa • 1 cup water • 1/2 cup black beans, drained and rinsed • 1/2 cup corn kernels • 1/2 cup diced tomatoes • 1/4 cup chopped cilantro • 1 teaspoon ground cumin • 1 teaspoon chili powder • Salt and pepper to taste

Instructions: Preheat the oven to 375°F (190°C). Rinse the quinoa under cold water. In a saucepan, bring 1 cup of water to a boil, add quinoa, reduce heat to low, cover, and simmer for 15 minutes, or until water is absorbed. In a large bowl, combine cooked quinoa, black beans, corn, diced tomatoes, cilantro, cumin, chili powder, salt, and pepper. Stuff the bell pepper halves with the quinoa mixture and place in a baking dish. Cover with foil and bake for 30 minutes, or until peppers are tender. Serve immediately.

Nutritional Information (per pepper): • Calories: 200 • Protein: 7g • Carbohydrates: 36g • Dietary Fiber: 10g • Fat: 3g • Saturated Fat: 0.5g • Sodium: 200mg • Potassium: 600mg • Phosphorus: 150mg

Turkey and Zucchini Meatballs

A lighter take on classic meatballs, these are perfect for a healthy dinner and pair well with pasta or salad.

Prep Time: 15 minutes

Cooking Time: 20 minutes

Serving Size: 4 meatballs (serves 2)

Ingredients: • 1/2 pound ground turkey • 1 small zucchini, grated • 1/4 cup breadcrumbs • 1 egg • 2 cloves garlic, minced • 1 teaspoon dried oregano • Salt and pepper to taste • 1 tablespoon olive oil

Instructions: Preheat the oven to 375°F (190°C). In a large bowl, combine ground turkey, grated zucchini, breadcrumbs, egg, garlic, oregano, salt, and pepper. Mix well and form into small meatballs. Heat olive oil in a large oven-safe skillet over medium heat. Add meatballs and cook until browned on all sides, about 5 minutes. Transfer the skillet to the oven and bake for 15 minutes, or until meatballs are cooked through. Serve immediately.

Nutritional Information (per serving): • Calories: 300 • Protein: 25g • Carbohydrates: 15g • Dietary Fiber: 2g • Fat: 15g • Saturated Fat: 3g • Sodium: 400mg • Potassium: 500mg • Phosphorus: 200mg

Baked Cod with Lemon and Garlic

A light and flavorful fish dish that's simple to prepare and perfect for a healthy dinner.

Prep Time: 10 minutes
Cooking Time: 20 minutes
Serving Size: 1 fillet (serves 2)

Ingredients: • 2 cod fillets • 2 tablespoons olive oil • Juice of 1 lemon • 2 cloves garlic, minced • 1 teaspoon dried parsley • Salt and pepper to taste

Instructions: Preheat the oven to 375°F (190°C). In a small bowl, whisk together olive oil, lemon juice, garlic, parsley, salt, and pepper. Place the cod fillets in a baking dish and pour the lemon garlic mixture over them. Bake for 20 minutes, or until the fish is opaque and flakes easily with a fork. Serve immediately.

Nutritional Information (per fillet): • Calories: 200 • Protein: 30g • Carbohydrates: 3g • Dietary Fiber: 0g • Fat: 8g • Saturated Fat: 1g • Sodium: 150mg • Potassium: 500mg • Phosphorus: 200mg

Vegetable Stir-Fry with Tofu

A quick and easy stir-fry that's packed with fresh vegetables and plant-based protein.

Prep Time: 10 minutes

Cooking Time: 10 minutes

Serving Size: 2 cups (serves 2)

Ingredients: • 1 block firm tofu, cubed • 1 cup broccoli florets • 1 bell pepper, sliced • 1 carrot, sliced • 2 tablespoons soy sauce • 1 tablespoon olive oil • 1 teaspoon grated ginger • 2 cloves garlic, minced

Instructions: Heat olive oil in a large skillet over medium-high heat. Add cubed tofu and cook until golden brown, about 5 minutes. Remove tofu from the skillet and set aside. Add broccoli, bell pepper, carrot, ginger, and garlic to the skillet. Stir-fry for about 5 minutes, or until vegetables are tender. Return tofu to the skillet, add soy sauce, and toss to combine. Serve immediately.

Nutritional Information (per cup): • Calories: 250 • Protein: 15g • Carbohydrates: 15g • Dietary Fiber: 5g •

Fat: 15g • Saturated Fat: 2g • Sodium: 500mg • Potassium: 500mg • Phosphorus: 250mg

Spinach and Mushroom Risotto

A creamy and delicious risotto that's full of flavor and perfect for a comforting dinner.

Prep Time: 10 minutes
Cooking Time: 30 minutes
Serving Size: 1 cup (serves 2)

Ingredients: • 1 cup Arborio rice • 1 tablespoon olive oil • 1 small onion, diced • 2 cloves garlic, minced • 1 cup sliced mushrooms • 4 cups low-sodium vegetable broth • 2 cups baby spinach • 1/4 cup grated Parmesan cheese (optional) • Salt and pepper to taste

Instructions: Heat olive oil in a large saucepan over medium heat. Add onion and garlic, cooking until softened. Add sliced mushrooms and cook until tender. Stir in Arborio rice and cook for 2 minutes, toasting the rice. Gradually add vegetable broth, one cup at a time, stirring frequently until absorbed before adding more. Continue until all broth is absorbed and rice is creamy and tender, about 20 minutes. Stir in baby spinach and cook until wilted. Season with salt and pepper and sprinkle with Parmesan cheese if desired. Serve immediately.

Nutritional Information (per cup): • Calories: 350 • Protein: 10g • Carbohydrates: 60g • Dietary Fiber: 4g • Fat: 10g • Saturated Fat: 2g • Sodium: 300mg • Potassium: 400mg • Phosphorus: 200mg

Chickpea and Spinach Curry

A hearty and flavorful curry that's rich in protein and perfect for a satisfying dinner.

Prep Time: 10 minutes
Cooking Time: 20 minutes
Serving Size: 1 cup (serves 2)

Ingredients: • 1 can chickpeas, drained and rinsed • 2 cups baby spinach • 1 small onion, diced • 2 cloves garlic, minced • 1 tablespoon olive oil • 1 tablespoon curry powder • 1 can diced tomatoes • 1/2 cup coconut milk • Salt and pepper to taste

Instructions: Heat olive oil in a large saucepan over medium heat. Add onion and garlic, cooking until softened. Stir in curry powder and cook for 1 minute, until fragrant. Add chickpeas, diced tomatoes, and coconut milk. Bring to a simmer and cook for 10 minutes, until the sauce has thickened. Stir in baby spinach and cook until wilted. Season with salt and pepper and serve immediately.

Nutritional Information (per cup): • Calories: 300 • Protein: 10g • Carbohydrates: 40g • Dietary Fiber: 10g • Fat: 12g • Saturated Fat: 6g • Sodium: 400mg • Potassium: 500mg • Phosphorus: 200mg

Beef and Vegetable Skewers

A delicious and healthy option for a main course, featuring lean beef and fresh vegetables.

Prep Time: 15 minutes
Cooking Time: 15 minutes
Serving Size: 2 skewers (serves 2)

Ingredients: • 1/2 pound lean beef, cut into cubes • 1 bell pepper, cut into chunks • 1 zucchini, sliced • 1 red onion, cut into chunks • 1 tablespoon olive oil • 2 tablespoons soy sauce • 1 teaspoon dried oregano • Salt and pepper to taste

Instructions: Preheat the grill to medium-high heat. In a large bowl, toss beef cubes, bell pepper, zucchini, and red onion with olive oil, soy sauce, oregano, salt, and pepper. Thread beef and vegetables onto skewers. Grill for about 10-15 minutes, turning occasionally, until beef is cooked to desired doneness and vegetables are tender. Serve immediately.

Nutritional Information (per skewer): • Calories: 250 • Protein: 20g • Carbohydrates: 10g • Dietary Fiber: 3g • Fat: 15g • Saturated Fat: 3g • Sodium: 500mg • Potassium: 500mg • Phosphorus: 200mg

ONE POT DINNER

Chicken and Vegetable Stir-Fry

A simple and delicious dinner option loaded with lean protein and colorful vegetables, perfect for a nutritious meal.

Prep Time: 15 minutes

Cooking Time: 20 minutes

Serving Size: 1 bowl

Ingredients:

- 1 chicken breast, thinly sliced
- 1 red bell pepper, sliced
- 1 yellow bell pepper, sliced
- 1 cup broccoli florets
- 1 carrot, julienned
- 2 tablespoons low-sodium soy sauce
- 1 tablespoon olive oil
- 2 cloves garlic, minced
- 1 teaspoon grated ginger
- 1 cup cooked brown rice

Instructions:

In a large skillet, heat olive oil over medium-high heat. Add garlic and ginger, sautéing until fragrant. Add chicken slices and cook until no longer pink, about 5-7 minutes. Add bell peppers, broccoli, and carrot, stirring to combine. Pour in soy sauce and cook until vegetables are tender-crisp, about 10 minutes. Serve over cooked brown rice.

Nutritional Information (per bowl):

• Calories: 350

• Protein: 30g

• Carbohydrates: 40g

• Dietary Fiber: 7g

• Fat: 10g

• Saturated Fat: 2g

• Sodium: 400mg

• Potassium: 800mg

• Phosphorus: 300mg

Lentil and Spinach Stew

This hearty stew is packed with fiber and protein, making it an excellent choice for a nourishing dinner.

Prep Time: 10 minutes
Cooking Time: 30 minutes
Serving Size: 1 bowl

Ingredients:

• 1 cup dried lentils

• 1 small onion, diced

• 2 cloves garlic, minced

• 1 carrot, diced

- 1 celery stalk, diced
- 1 can diced tomatoes
- 4 cups vegetable broth
- 2 cups baby spinach
- 1 tablespoon olive oil
- 1 teaspoon cumin
- Salt and pepper to taste

Instructions:

In a large pot, heat olive oil over medium heat. Add onion, garlic, carrot, and celery, cooking until softened. Add lentils, diced tomatoes, vegetable broth, and cumin. Bring to a boil, then reduce heat and simmer for 25 minutes or until lentils are tender. Stir in baby spinach and cook until wilted. Season with salt and pepper and serve hot.

Nutritional Information (per bowl):

- Calories: 300
- Protein: 18g
- Carbohydrates: 50g
- Dietary Fiber: 16g
- Fat: 6g
- Saturated Fat: 1g
- Sodium: 500mg

- Potassium: 900mg
- Phosphorus: 350mg

Shrimp and Quinoa Paella

A light and flavorful dish inspired by traditional paella, featuring shrimp and quinoa for a healthy twist.

Prep Time: 10 minutes
Cooking Time: 25 minutes
Serving Size: 1 bowl

Ingredients:
- 1/2 cup quinoa, rinsed
- 1/2 pound shrimp, peeled and deveined
- 1/2 red bell pepper, diced
- 1/2 green bell pepper, diced
- 1 small onion, diced
- 1 clove garlic, minced
- 1 cup low-sodium chicken broth
- 1/2 cup diced tomatoes
- 1 teaspoon smoked paprika
- 1 tablespoon olive oil
- Salt and pepper to taste

Instructions:

In a large skillet, heat olive oil over medium heat. Add onion, garlic, and bell peppers, cooking until softened. Add quinoa, diced tomatoes, chicken broth, and smoked paprika. Bring to a boil, then reduce heat and simmer for 15 minutes. Add shrimp and cook until pink and opaque, about 5-7 minutes. Season with salt and pepper and serve immediately.

Nutritional Information (per bowl):
• Calories: 350
• Protein: 25g
• Carbohydrates: 45g
• Dietary Fiber: 6g
• Fat: 9g
• Saturated Fat: 1g
• Sodium: 400mg
• Potassium: 600mg
• Phosphorus: 300mg

Turkey and Sweet Potato Skillet

A comforting and nutritious one-pot meal featuring lean turkey and sweet potatoes, perfect for a cozy dinner.

Prep Time: 10 minutes
Cooking Time: 25 minutes
Serving Size: 1 bowl

Ingredients:

- 1/2 pound ground turkey
- 1 large sweet potato, diced
- 1 small onion, diced
- 1 bell pepper, diced
- 2 cloves garlic, minced
- 1 cup baby spinach
- 1 teaspoon ground cumin
- 1 teaspoon paprika
- 1 tablespoon olive oil
- Salt and pepper to taste

Instructions:

In a large skillet, heat olive oil over medium heat. Add onion and garlic, cooking until softened. Add ground turkey, breaking it up with a spoon, and cook until no longer pink. Add sweet potato, bell pepper, cumin, and paprika, stirring to combine. Cover and cook for 15 minutes or until sweet potatoes are tender. Stir in baby spinach and cook until wilted. Season with salt and pepper and serve immediately.

Nutritional Information (per bowl):

- Calories: 400
- Protein: 28g
- Carbohydrates: 50g
- Dietary Fiber: 8g
- Fat: 12g
- Saturated Fat: 2g
- Sodium: 350mg
- Potassium: 1000mg
- Phosphorus: 350mg

Vegetable and Tofu Stir-Fry

A light and healthy option featuring a mix of fresh vegetables and tofu, perfect for a quick dinner.

Prep Time: 15 minutes

Cooking Time: 20 minutes

Serving Size: 1 bowl

Ingredients:

- 1 block firm tofu, pressed and cubed
- 1 cup broccoli florets
- 1 carrot, julienned
- 1 bell pepper, sliced
- 1 small onion, sliced
- 2 tablespoons low-sodium soy sauce
- 1 tablespoon olive oil
- 1 clove garlic, minced
- 1 teaspoon grated ginger
- 1 cup cooked brown rice

Instructions:

In a large skillet, heat olive oil over medium-high heat. Add garlic and ginger, sautéing until fragrant. Add tofu cubes and cook until golden brown, about 5-7 minutes. Add broccoli, carrot, bell pepper, and onion, stirring to combine. Pour in soy sauce and cook until vegetables are tender-crisp, about 10 minutes. Serve over cooked brown rice.

Nutritional Information (per bowl):

- Calories: 350
- Protein: 20g
- Carbohydrates: 40g

- Dietary Fiber: 8g

- Fat: 12g

- Saturated Fat: 2g

- Sodium: 400mg

- Potassium: 800mg

- Phosphorus: 300mg

Quinoa and Black Bean Chili

A hearty and filling chili made with quinoa and black beans, perfect for a comforting dinner.

Prep Time: 10 minutes
Cooking Time: 30 minutes
Serving Size: 1 bowl

Ingredients:
- 1/2 cup quinoa, rinsed

- 1 can black beans, drained and rinsed

- 1 can diced tomatoes

- 1 small onion, diced

- 1 bell pepper, diced

- 2 cloves garlic, minced

- 1 tablespoon chili powder

- 1 teaspoon cumin

- 4 cups vegetable broth
- 1 tablespoon olive oil
- Salt and pepper to taste

Instructions:

In a large pot, heat olive oil over medium heat. Add onion, garlic, and bell pepper, cooking until softened. Add quinoa, black beans, diced tomatoes, vegetable broth, chili powder, and cumin. Bring to a boil, then reduce heat and simmer for 25 minutes or until quinoa is tender. Season with salt and pepper and serve hot.

Nutritional Information (per bowl):

- Calories: 350
- Protein: 15g
- Carbohydrates: 55g
- Dietary Fiber: 15g
- Fat: 8g
- Saturated Fat: 1g
- Sodium: 500mg
- Potassium: 900mg
- Phosphorus: 300mg

Chicken and Rice Casserole

A classic casserole dish made healthier with brown rice and lean chicken, ideal for a satisfying dinner.

Prep Time: 10 minutes
Cooking Time: 30 minutes
Serving Size: 1 bowl

Ingredients:

- 1 chicken breast, diced
- 1 cup brown rice
- 1 cup broccoli florets
- 1 small onion, diced
- 2 cloves garlic, minced
- 2 cups low-sodium chicken broth
- 1/2 cup low-fat milk
- 1 tablespoon olive oil
- Salt and pepper to taste

Instructions:

In a large pot, heat olive oil over medium heat. Add onion and garlic, cooking until softened. Add diced chicken and cook until no longer pink. Stir in brown rice, broccoli, chicken broth, and low-fat milk. Bring to a boil, then reduce heat and simmer for 25 minutes or until rice is tender and liquid is absorbed. Season with salt and pepper and serve immediately.

Nutritional Information (per bowl):
• Calories: 400
• Protein: 30g
• Carbohydrates: 50g
• Dietary Fiber: 5g
• Fat: 10g
• Saturated Fat: 2g
• Sodium: 400mg
• Potassium: 800mg
• Phosphorus: 300mg

Beef and Vegetable Stew

A robust and flavorful stew made with lean beef and a variety of vegetables, perfect for a hearty dinner.

Prep Time: 15 minutes
Cooking Time: 45 minutes
Serving Size: 1 bowl

Ingredients:

• 1/2 pound lean beef stew meat, cubed

• 1 large potato, diced

• 1 carrot, sliced

• 1 celery stalk, sliced

• 1 small onion, diced

• 2 cloves garlic, minced

• 1 can diced tomatoes

• 4 cups low-sodium beef broth

• 1 tablespoon olive oil

• Salt and pepper to taste

Instructions:

In a large pot, heat olive oil over medium heat. Add onion and garlic, cooking until softened. Add beef cubes and cook until browned on all sides. Add potato, carrot, celery, diced tomatoes, and beef broth. Bring to a boil, then reduce heat and simmer for 40 minutes or until vegetables are tender and beef is cooked through. Season with salt and pepper and serve hot.

Nutritional Information (per bowl):

• Calories: 450

• Protein: 30g

• Carbohydrates: 40g

- Dietary Fiber: 7g
- Fat: 15g
- Saturated Fat: 4g
- Sodium: 500mg
- Potassium: 1000mg
- Phosphorus: 350mg

Mushroom and Barley Soup

A comforting soup made with mushrooms and barley, perfect for a warm and filling dinner.

Prep Time: 10 minutes
Cooking Time: 30 minutes
Serving Size: 1 bowl

Ingredients:
- 1 cup sliced mushrooms
- 1/2 cup pearl barley
- 1 small onion, diced
- 2 cloves garlic, minced
- 1 carrot, diced
- 4 cups vegetable broth
- 1 tablespoon olive oil

- 1 teaspoon thyme
- Salt and pepper to taste

Instructions:

In a large pot, heat olive oil over medium heat. Add onion, garlic, and carrot, cooking until softened. Add mushrooms and cook until tender. Stir in barley, vegetable broth, and thyme. Bring to a boil, then reduce heat and simmer for 30 minutes or until barley is tender. Season with salt and pepper and serve hot.

Nutritional Information (per bowl):

- Calories: 300
- Protein: 8g
- Carbohydrates: 55g
- Dietary Fiber: 10g
- Fat: 7g
- Saturated Fat: 1g
- Sodium: 400mg
- Potassium: 700mg
- Phosphorus: 200mg

Mediterranean Chickpea Stew

A flavorful stew featuring chickpeas and Mediterranean spices, perfect for a quick and healthy dinner.

Prep Time: 10 minutes
Cooking Time: 25 minutes
Serving Size: 1 bowl

Ingredients:

- 1 can chickpeas, drained and rinsed
- 1 can diced tomatoes
- 1 small onion, diced
- 2 cloves garlic, minced
- 1 bell pepper, diced
- 1 zucchini, sliced
- 1 tablespoon olive oil
- 1 teaspoon ground cumin
- 1 teaspoon paprika
- 4 cups vegetable broth
- Salt and pepper to taste

Instructions:

In a large pot, heat olive oil over medium heat. Add onion, garlic, and bell pepper, cooking until softened.

Add chickpeas, diced tomatoes, zucchini, vegetable broth, cumin, and paprika. Bring to a boil, then reduce heat and simmer for 20 minutes or until vegetables are tender. Season with salt and pepper and serve hot.

Nutritional Information (per bowl):
- Calories: 350
- Protein: 12g
- Carbohydrates: 60g
- Dietary Fiber: 14g
- Fat: 9g
- Saturated Fat: 1g
- Sodium: 500mg
- Potassium: 800mg
- Phosphorus: 250mg

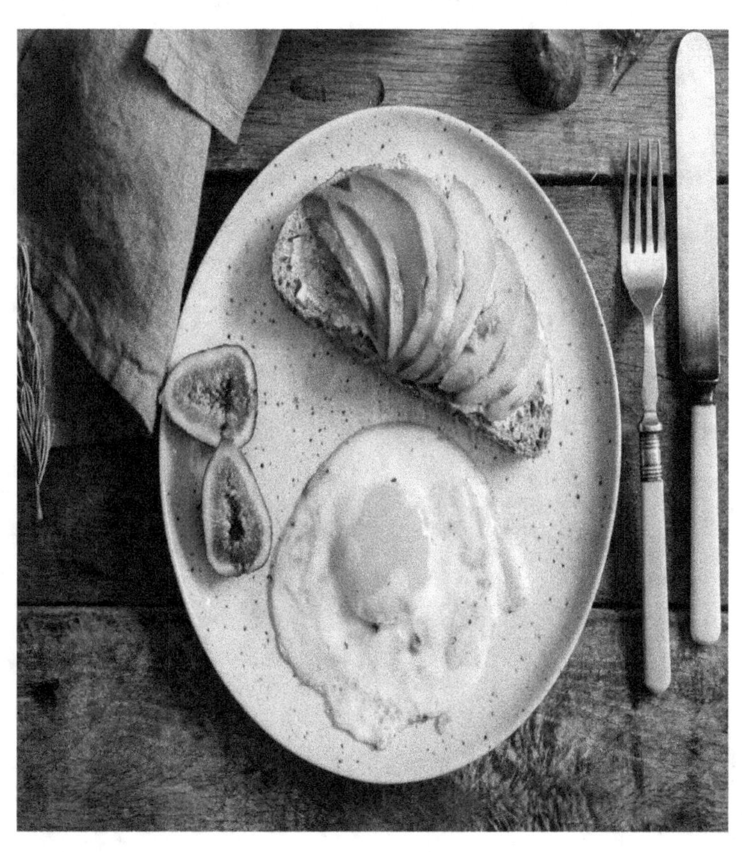

CHAPTER 7: SNACKS AND APPETIZERS

Healthy Snacking Options

Hummus and Veggie Sticks

A nutritious and satisfying snack packed with protein and fiber, perfect for a quick and healthy bite.

Prep Time: 10 minutes
Cooking Time: 0 minutes
Serving Size: 1 cup

Ingredients:
- 1 cup canned chickpeas, drained and rinsed
- 2 tablespoons tahini
- 1 tablespoon olive oil
- 1 clove garlic, minced
- Juice of 1 lemon
- 1/4 teaspoon ground cumin
- Salt and pepper to taste
- 1 carrot, cut into sticks

- 1 cucumber, cut into sticks
- 1 bell pepper, cut into sticks

Instructions:

In a food processor, combine chickpeas, tahini, olive oil, garlic, lemon juice, and cumin. Blend until smooth, adding a tablespoon of water if needed for a creamier consistency. Season with salt and pepper to taste. Serve hummus with carrot, cucumber, and bell pepper sticks.

Nutritional Information (per cup):
- Calories: 250
- Protein: 7g
- Carbohydrates: 29g
- Dietary Fiber: 9g
- Fat: 12g
- Saturated Fat: 2g
- Sodium: 180mg
- Potassium: 400mg
- Phosphorus: 120mg

Greek Yogurt with Berries

A refreshing and protein-rich snack that is both delicious and easy to prepare.

Prep Time: 5 minutes

Cooking Time: 0 minutes

Serving Size: 1 cup

Ingredients:

• 1 cup low-fat Greek yogurt

• 1/2 cup mixed berries (strawberries, blueberries, raspberries)

• 1 teaspoon honey (optional)

• 1 tablespoon chia seeds

Instructions:

In a bowl, combine Greek yogurt and mixed berries. Drizzle with honey if desired and sprinkle with chia seeds. Mix gently and serve immediately.

Nutritional Information (per cup):

• Calories: 180

• Protein: 15g

• Carbohydrates: 22g

• Dietary Fiber: 6g

• Fat: 4g

• Saturated Fat: 1g

• Sodium: 60mg

- Potassium: 300mg
- Phosphorus: 180mg

Apple Slices with Peanut Butter

A classic and satisfying snack that pairs the sweetness of apples with the richness of peanut butter.

Prep Time: 5 minutes
Cooking Time: 0 minutes
Serving Size: 1 cup

Ingredients:
- 1 large apple, sliced
- 2 tablespoons natural peanut butter

Instructions:
Core and slice the apple into wedges. Serve with a side of natural peanut butter for dipping.

Nutritional Information (per cup):
- Calories: 200
- Protein: 4g
- Carbohydrates: 28g
- Dietary Fiber: 5g
- Fat: 8g

- Saturated Fat: 1g

- Sodium: 2mg

- Potassium: 300mg

- Phosphorus: 70mg

Roasted Chickpeas

A crunchy and savory snack that is high in protein and fiber, perfect for munching.

Prep Time: 5 minutes

Cooking Time: 30 minutes

Serving Size: 1 cup

Ingredients:

- 1 cup canned chickpeas, drained and rinsed

- 1 tablespoon olive oil

- 1 teaspoon paprika

- 1/2 teaspoon garlic powder

- Salt and pepper to taste

Instructions:

Preheat oven to 400°F (200°C). Pat chickpeas dry with a paper towel. In a bowl, toss chickpeas with olive oil, paprika, garlic powder, salt, and pepper. Spread chickpeas on a baking sheet in a single layer. Roast for 30 minutes, shaking the pan halfway through, until chickpeas are crispy. Allow to cool before serving.

Nutritional Information (per cup):

- Calories: 200
- Protein: 8g
- Carbohydrates: 30g
- Dietary Fiber: 9g
- Fat: 8g
- Saturated Fat: 1g
- Sodium: 200mg
- Potassium: 300mg
- Phosphorus: 120mg

Cottage Cheese with Pineapple

A refreshing and protein-packed snack that combines the creaminess of cottage cheese with the sweetness of pineapple.

Prep Time: 5 minutes
Cooking Time: 0 minutes
Serving Size: 1 cup

Ingredients:

- 1 cup low-fat cottage cheese
- 1/2 cup pineapple chunks (fresh or canned in juice)

Instructions:

In a bowl, combine low-fat cottage cheese and pineapple chunks. Mix gently and serve immediately.

Nutritional Information (per cup):

- Calories: 180
- Protein: 16g
- Carbohydrates: 20g
- Dietary Fiber: 2g
- Fat: 4g
- Saturated Fat: 2g
- Sodium: 400mg
- Potassium: 300mg
- Phosphorus: 200mg

Edamame with Sea Salt

A simple and nutritious snack that is high in protein and fiber, great for a quick and healthy bite.

Prep Time: 5 minutes

Cooking Time: 5 minutes

Serving Size: 1 cup

Ingredients:

• 1 cup frozen edamame in pods

• 1/4 teaspoon sea salt

Instructions:

Bring a pot of water to a boil. Add edamame and cook for 5 minutes. Drain and sprinkle with sea salt. Serve warm or cold.

Nutritional Information (per cup):

• Calories: 190

• Protein: 17g

• Carbohydrates: 14g

• Dietary Fiber: 8g

• Fat: 8g

• Saturated Fat: 1g

• Sodium: 180mg

• Potassium: 540mg

• Phosphorus: 240mg

Banana and Oat Energy Bites

A quick and easy snack that is perfect for on-the-go energy, made with simple and wholesome ingredients.

Prep Time: 10 minutes
Cooking Time: 0 minutes
Serving Size: 1 cup

Ingredients:
- 1 ripe banana, mashed
- 1 cup rolled oats
- 2 tablespoons natural peanut butter
- 1 tablespoon honey
- 1 teaspoon vanilla extract

Instructions:
In a bowl, combine mashed banana, rolled oats, peanut butter, honey, and vanilla extract. Mix until well combined. Roll the mixture into small balls. Refrigerate for at least 30 minutes before serving.

Nutritional Information (per cup):
- Calories: 220
- Protein: 6g

- Carbohydrates: 36g
- Dietary Fiber: 5g
- Fat: 7g
- Saturated Fat: 1g
- Sodium: 20mg
- Potassium: 300mg
- Phosphorus: 100mg

Avocado and Tomato Toast

A delicious and heart-healthy snack that is both flavorful and filling, perfect for a light bite.

Prep Time: 5 minutes
Cooking Time: 5 minutes
Serving Size: 1 cup

Ingredients:
- 1 avocado, mashed
- 1 small tomato, sliced
- 2 slices whole grain bread
- Salt and pepper to taste
- 1 teaspoon lemon juice

Instructions:

Toast the bread slices until golden brown. Spread mashed avocado on each slice. Top with tomato slices, sprinkle with salt and pepper, and drizzle with lemon juice. Serve immediately.

Nutritional Information (per cup):

- Calories: 250
- Protein: 6g
- Carbohydrates: 28g
- Dietary Fiber: 10g
- Fat: 15g
- Saturated Fat: 2g
- Sodium: 180mg
- Potassium: 700mg
- Phosphorus: 100mg

Greek Yogurt with Cucumber and Mint

A refreshing and creamy snack that is both light and satisfying, ideal for a quick pick-me-up.

Prep Time: 5 minutes

Cooking Time: 0 minutes

Serving Size: 1 cup

Ingredients:

- 1 cup low-fat Greek yogurt
- 1/2 cucumber, diced
- 1 tablespoon fresh mint, chopped
- 1 teaspoon lemon juice
- Salt and pepper to taste

Instructions:

In a bowl, combine Greek yogurt, diced cucumber, chopped mint, and lemon juice. Mix well and season with salt and pepper. Serve chilled.

Nutritional Information (per cup):

- Calories: 120
- Protein: 15g
- Carbohydrates: 8g
- Dietary Fiber: 1g
- Fat: 4g
- Saturated Fat: 2g
- Sodium: 70mg

- Potassium: 300mg
- Phosphorus: 180mg

Celery Sticks with Hummus

A crunchy and flavorful snack that is easy to prepare and packed with nutrients, perfect for a healthy treat.

Prep Time: 5 minutes
Cooking Time: 0 minutes
Serving Size: 1 cup

Ingredients:
- 4 celery sticks, cut into 3-inch pieces
- 1/2 cup hummus (store-bought or homemade)

Instructions:
Arrange celery sticks on a plate. Serve with a side of hummus for dipping.

Nutritional Information (per cup):
- Calories: 150
- Protein: 4g
- Carbohydrates: 20g
- Dietary Fiber: 6g
- Fat: 8g

- Saturated Fat: 1g
- Sodium: 250mg
- Potassium: 300mg
- Phosphorus: 100mg

Easy-to-Prepare Appetizers

Cucumber and Hummus Bites

A light and refreshing appetizer that is both healthy and easy to prepare, perfect for a quick snack or party starter.

Prep Time: 10 minutes
Cooking Time: 0 minutes
Serving Size: 1 cup

Ingredients:
- 1 cucumber, sliced into rounds
- 1/2 cup hummus
- 1 tablespoon chopped fresh dill
- 1 teaspoon lemon zest
- Salt and pepper to taste

Instructions:

Arrange cucumber slices on a serving platter. Top each slice with a dollop of hummus. Sprinkle with chopped dill and lemon zest. Season with salt and pepper to taste. Serve immediately.

Nutritional Information (per cup):

- Calories: 80
- Protein: 3g
- Carbohydrates: 12g
- Dietary Fiber: 3g
- Fat: 3g
- Saturated Fat: 0.5g
- Sodium: 140mg
- Potassium: 250mg
- Phosphorus: 50mg

Caprese Skewers

A classic Italian appetizer that is simple, flavorful, and healthy, featuring fresh tomatoes, mozzarella, and basil.

Prep Time: 10 minutes

Cooking Time: 0 minutes

Serving Size: 1 cup

Ingredients:

- 10 cherry tomatoes
- 10 small mozzarella balls (bocconcini)
- 10 fresh basil leaves
- 1 tablespoon balsamic glaze
- 1 teaspoon olive oil
- Salt and pepper to taste

Instructions:

Thread one cherry tomato, one mozzarella ball, and one basil leaf onto each skewer. Arrange skewers on a serving platter. Drizzle with balsamic glaze and olive oil. Season with salt and pepper to taste. Serve immediately.

Nutritional Information (per cup):

- Calories: 120
- Protein: 7g
- Carbohydrates: 6g
- Dietary Fiber: 1g
- Fat: 8g
- Saturated Fat: 3g
- Sodium: 150mg
- Potassium: 200mg
- Phosphorus: 100mg

Avocado and Black Bean Salsa

A vibrant and nutritious appetizer that combines the creamy texture of avocado with the protein-rich black beans, perfect for dipping or as a topping. Prep Time: 10 minutes

Cooking Time: 0 minutes

Serving Size: 1 cup

Ingredients:

- 1 avocado, diced
- 1/2 cup canned black beans, drained and rinsed
- 1/2 cup diced tomatoes
- 1/4 cup chopped red onion
- 1 tablespoon chopped fresh cilantro
- Juice of 1 lime
- Salt and pepper to taste

Instructions:

In a bowl, combine diced avocado, black beans, tomatoes, red onion, and cilantro. Squeeze lime juice over the mixture and stir gently to combine. Season with salt and pepper to taste. Serve immediately.

Nutritional Information (per cup):

• Calories: 200

• Protein: 5g

• Carbohydrates: 20g

• Dietary Fiber: 9g

• Fat: 13g

• Saturated Fat: 2g

• Sodium: 150mg

• Potassium: 650mg

• Phosphorus: 100mg

Greek Yogurt and Herb Dip

A creamy and tangy dip made with Greek yogurt and fresh herbs, perfect for pairing with vegetable sticks or whole-grain crackers. Prep Time: 5 minutes
Cooking Time: 0 minutes
Serving Size: 1 cup

Ingredients:

• 1 cup low-fat Greek yogurt

• 1 tablespoon chopped fresh parsley

• 1 tablespoon chopped fresh dill

• 1 clove garlic, minced

- Juice of 1/2 lemon

- Salt and pepper to taste

Instructions:

In a bowl, combine Greek yogurt, parsley, dill, minced garlic, and lemon juice. Stir until well mixed. Season with salt and pepper to taste. Serve immediately with vegetable sticks or whole-grain crackers.

Nutritional Information (per cup):

- Calories: 100

- Protein: 10g

- Carbohydrates: 7g

- Dietary Fiber: 0g

- Fat: 3g

- Saturated Fat: 2g

- Sodium: 70mg

- Potassium: 200mg

- Phosphorus: 140mg

Tomato Basil Bruschetta

A flavorful and easy-to-make appetizer that features fresh tomatoes, basil, and garlic on toasted baguette slices. Prep Time: 10 minutes

Cooking Time: 5 minutes

Serving Size: 1 cup

Ingredients:

- 1 baguette, sliced into rounds
- 2 tomatoes, diced
- 1 tablespoon chopped fresh basil
- 1 clove garlic, minced
- 1 tablespoon olive oil
- Salt and pepper to taste

Instructions:

Preheat the oven to 400°F (200°C). Arrange baguette slices on a baking sheet and toast for 5 minutes or until golden brown. In a bowl, combine diced tomatoes, basil, garlic, and olive oil. Season with salt and pepper to taste. Spoon the tomato mixture onto the toasted baguette slices and serve immediately.

Nutritional Information (per cup):

- Calories: 150
- Protein: 4g
- Carbohydrates: 22g
- Dietary Fiber: 2g
- Fat: 6g

- Saturated Fat: 1g
- Sodium: 250mg
- Potassium: 250mg
- Phosphorus: 60mg

Stuffed Mini Bell Peppers

A colorful and nutritious appetizer that is easy to make and full of flavor, featuring mini bell peppers stuffed with a creamy cheese mixture. Prep Time: 10 minutes Cooking Time: 0 minutes Serving Size: 1 cup

Ingredients:

- 10 mini bell peppers, halved and seeded
- 1/2 cup low-fat cream cheese
- 1/4 cup crumbled feta cheese
- 1 tablespoon chopped fresh parsley
- 1 teaspoon lemon zest
- Salt and pepper to taste

Instructions:

In a bowl, combine cream cheese, feta cheese, parsley, and lemon zest. Season with salt and pepper to taste.

Spoon the cheese mixture into the halved bell peppers. Arrange on a serving platter and serve immediately.

Nutritional Information (per cup):

• Calories: 120

• Protein: 5g

• Carbohydrates: 10g

• Dietary Fiber: 2g

• Fat: 8g

• Saturated Fat: 4g

• Sodium: 250mg

• Potassium: 250mg

• Phosphorus: 100mg

Spinach and Feta Stuffed Mushrooms

A savory appetizer that is both delicious and healthy, featuring mushrooms stuffed with a flavorful spinach and feta mixture. Prep Time: 10 minutes
Cooking Time: 20 minutes
Serving Size: 1 cup

Ingredients:
• 10 large mushrooms, stems removed
• 1 cup fresh spinach, chopped

- 1/4 cup crumbled feta cheese

- 1 clove garlic, minced

- 1 tablespoon olive oil

- Salt and pepper to taste

Instructions:

Preheat the oven to 375°F (190°C). In a skillet, heat olive oil over medium heat. Add garlic and spinach, and cook until spinach is wilted. Remove from heat and stir in feta cheese. Season with salt and pepper to taste. Spoon the mixture into the mushroom caps and arrange on a baking sheet. Bake for 20 minutes or until mushrooms are tender. Serve immediately.

Nutritional Information (per cup):

- Calories: 100

- Protein: 5g

- Carbohydrates: 5g

- Dietary Fiber: 2g

- Fat: 7g

- Saturated Fat: 2g

- Sodium: 220mg

- Potassium: 300mg

- Phosphorus: 80mg

Zucchini Fritters

A light and crispy appetizer that is easy to prepare and packed with vegetables, perfect for a healthy snack or starter.

Prep Time: 10 minutes
Cooking Time: 10 minutes
Serving Size: 1 cup

Ingredients:
- 1 medium zucchini, grated
- 1/4 cup whole wheat flour
- 1 egg, beaten
- 1 clove garlic, minced
- 1 tablespoon chopped fresh dill
- Salt and pepper to taste
- 1 tablespoon olive oil

Instructions:
In a bowl, combine grated zucchini, whole wheat flour, beaten egg, garlic, dill, salt, and pepper. Mix well. Heat olive oil in a skillet over medium heat. Drop spoonfuls of the zucchini mixture into the skillet and flatten slightly.

Cook for 3-4 minutes on each side until golden brown. Drain on paper towels and serve immediately.

Nutritional Information (per cup):

• Calories: 150

• Protein: 6g

• Carbohydrates: 16g

• Dietary Fiber: 3g

• Fat: 8g

• Saturated Fat: 1g

• Sodium: 150mg

• Potassium: 400mg

• Phosphorus: 70mg

Carrot and Cucumber Rolls

A fresh and crunchy appetizer that is easy to make and full of flavor, featuring thinly sliced vegetables rolled with a creamy filling. Prep Time: 10 minutes
Cooking Time: 0 minutes
Serving Size: 1 cup

Ingredients:

• 1 carrot, thinly sliced

• 1 cucumber, thinly sliced

- 1/4 cup low-fat cream cheese
- 1 tablespoon chopped fresh chives
- 1 teaspoon lemon zest
- Salt and pepper to taste

Instructions:

In a bowl, combine cream cheese, chives, and lemon zest. Season with salt and pepper to taste. Spread a thin layer of the cream cheese mixture on each slice of carrot and cucumber. Roll up each slice and secure with a toothpick if necessary. Arrange on a serving platter and serve immediately.

Nutritional Information (per cup):

- Calories: 80
- Protein: 3g
- Carbohydrates: 10g
- Dietary Fiber: 2g
- Fat: 3g
- Saturated Fat: 1.5g
- Sodium: 100mg
- Potassium: 300mg
- Phosphorus: 50mg

Chickpea and Avocado Toast

A nutritious and filling appetizer that combines creamy avocado with protein-rich chickpeas on whole grain toast.

Prep Time: 10 minutes
Cooking Time: 0 minutes
Serving Size: 1 cup

Ingredients:

- 2 slices whole grain bread, toasted
- 1/2 avocado, mashed
- 1/2 cup canned chickpeas, drained and rinsed
- 1 tablespoon lemon juice
- Salt and pepper to taste

Instructions:

In a bowl, combine mashed avocado, chickpeas, and lemon juice. Season with salt and pepper to taste. Spread the mixture evenly over the toasted whole grain bread slices. Cut each slice in half and serve immediately.

Nutritional Information (per cup):

• Calories: 250

• Protein: 8g

• Carbohydrates: 35g

• Dietary Fiber: 9g

• Fat: 10g

• Saturated Fat: 1.5g

• Sodium: 150mg

• Potassium: 450mg

• Phosphorus: 120mg

Beet and Goat Cheese Salad

A vibrant and flavorful appetizer that combines sweet beets with tangy goat cheese, perfect for a light and healthy starter.

Prep Time: 10 minutes
Cooking Time: 30 minutes
Serving Size: 1 cup

Ingredients:

• 2 medium beets, roasted and diced

• 1/4 cup crumbled goat cheese

• 1 tablespoon balsamic vinegar

- 1 tablespoon olive oil

- 1 tablespoon chopped fresh parsley

- Salt and pepper to taste

Instructions:

Preheat the oven to 375°F (190°C). Wrap beets in aluminum foil and roast for 30 minutes or until tender. Let cool, then dice. In a bowl, combine diced beets, goat cheese, balsamic vinegar, olive oil, and parsley. Season with salt and pepper to taste. Toss gently and serve immediately.

Nutritional Information (per cup):

- Calories: 180

- Protein: 5g

- Carbohydrates: 16g

- Dietary Fiber: 4g

- Fat: 12g

- Saturated Fat: 4g

- Sodium: 150mg

- Potassium: 400mg

- Phosphorus: 100mg

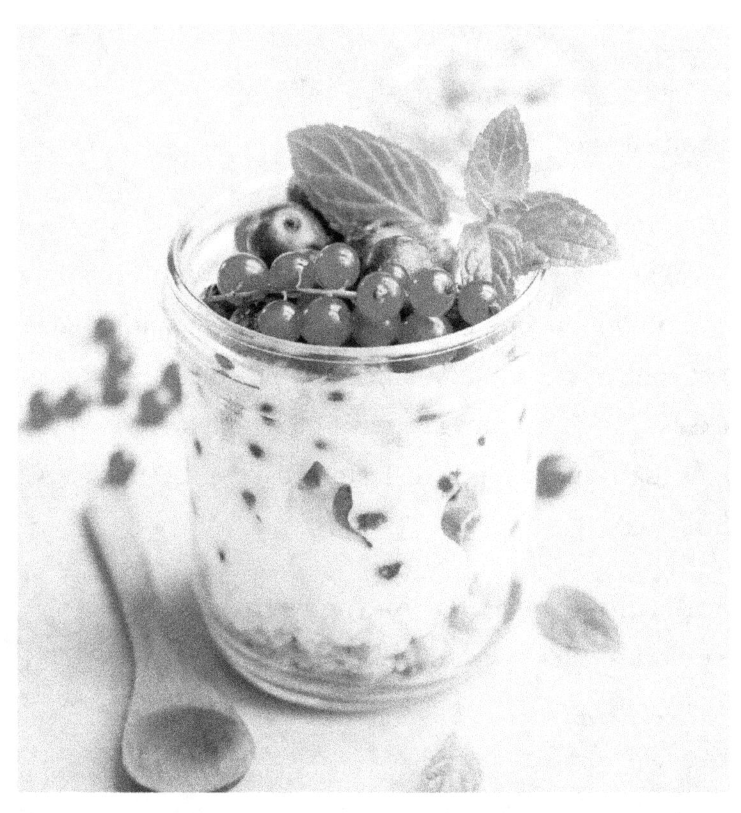

Chapter 8: Desserts and Treats

Low-Fat Sweet Treats

Berry Yogurt Parfait

A delicious and refreshing dessert that combines creamy yogurt with fresh berries and a hint of honey.

Prep Time: 5 minutes
Cooking Time: 0 minutes
Serving Size: 1 cup

Ingredients:

• 1 cup low-fat Greek yogurt

• 1/2 cup mixed berries (strawberries, blueberries, raspberries)

• 1 tablespoon honey

• 1 tablespoon granola (optional)

Instructions:

In a bowl or glass, layer half of the Greek yogurt. Top with half of the mixed berries. Repeat the layers with the remaining yogurt and berries. Drizzle with honey and sprinkle with granola if desired. Serve immediately.

Nutritional Information (per cup):

• Calories: 180

• Protein: 12g

• Carbohydrates: 30g

• Dietary Fiber: 4g

• Fat: 2g

• Saturated Fat: 0.5g

• Sodium: 70mg

• Potassium: 350mg

• Phosphorus: 150mg

Chocolate Banana Ice Cream

A creamy and guilt-free ice cream alternative made with frozen bananas and a touch of cocoa. Prep Time: 5 minutes
Cooking Time: 0 minutes
Serving Size: 1 cup

Ingredients:

• 2 ripe bananas, sliced and frozen

• 1 tablespoon unsweetened cocoa powder

• 1 teaspoon vanilla extract

Instructions:

Place the frozen banana slices in a food processor. Blend until smooth and creamy. Add cocoa powder and vanilla extract, and blend again until well combined. Serve immediately as soft-serve or freeze for an hour for a firmer texture.

Nutritional Information (per cup):

• Calories: 150

• Protein: 2g

• Carbohydrates: 38g

• Dietary Fiber: 4g

• Fat: 0.5g

• Saturated Fat: 0g

• Sodium: 1mg

• Potassium: 500mg

• Phosphorus: 25mg

Apple Cinnamon Baked Chips

A healthy and crunchy snack made from fresh apples with a hint of cinnamon, perfect for satisfying a sweet tooth.

Prep Time: 10 minutes
Cooking Time: 2 hours
Serving Size: 1 cup

Ingredients:
• 2 apples, thinly sliced
• 1/2 teaspoon ground cinnamon

Instructions:
Preheat the oven to 200°F (93°C). Arrange the apple slices in a single layer on a baking sheet lined with parchment paper. Sprinkle with ground cinnamon. Bake for 2 hours, flipping halfway through, until the apples are crisp. Let cool before serving.

Nutritional Information (per cup):
• Calories: 90
• Protein: 0g
• Carbohydrates: 24g
• Dietary Fiber: 4g
• Fat: 0g

- Saturated Fat: 0g
- Sodium: 0mg
- Potassium: 200mg
- Phosphorus: 20mg

Strawberry Banana Smoothie

A refreshing and nutritious smoothie that combines the sweetness of strawberries with the creaminess of bananas.

Prep Time: 5 minutes
Cooking Time: 0 minutes
Serving Size: 1 cup

Ingredients:
- 1 banana, sliced
- 1/2 cup strawberries, hulled
- 1/2 cup low-fat milk
- 1 teaspoon honey (optional)

Instructions:
In a blender, combine the banana, strawberries, and low-fat milk. Blend until smooth. Add honey if desired for extra sweetness. Serve immediately.

Nutritional Information (per cup):

• Calories: 150

• Protein: 4g

• Carbohydrates: 34g

• Dietary Fiber: 4g

• Fat: 1g

• Saturated Fat: 0.5g

• Sodium: 40mg

• Potassium: 500mg

• Phosphorus: 90mg

Blueberry Chia Pudding

A healthy and filling pudding made with chia seeds and fresh blueberries, perfect for a sweet treat or breakfast.

Prep Time: 5 minutes

Cooking Time: 0 minutes

Serving Size: 1 cup

Ingredients:

• 1/4 cup chia seeds

• 1 cup low-fat milk

• 1/2 cup blueberries

• 1 tablespoon honey

Instructions:

In a bowl, combine chia seeds and low-fat milk. Stir well and let sit for 5 minutes. Stir again to prevent clumping. Refrigerate for at least 4 hours or overnight. Before serving, top with blueberries and drizzle with honey.

Nutritional Information (per cup):

- Calories: 250
- Protein: 8g
- Carbohydrates: 30g
- Dietary Fiber: 12g
- Fat: 10g
- Saturated Fat: 1g
- Sodium: 50mg
- Potassium: 400mg
- Phosphorus: 200mg

Mango Sorbet

A refreshing and naturally sweet sorbet made with ripe mangoes, perfect for a light and fruity dessert.

Prep Time: 10 minutes

Cooking Time: 0 minutes

Serving Size: 1 cup

Ingredients:

• 2 ripe mangoes, peeled and chopped

• 1 tablespoon lime juice

• 1 teaspoon honey (optional)

Instructions:

In a blender, combine the mangoes, lime juice, and honey if using. Blend until smooth. Pour the mixture into a shallow container and freeze for at least 4 hours. Before serving, let the sorbet sit at room temperature for 5 minutes to soften slightly.

Nutritional Information (per cup):

• Calories: 120

• Protein: 1g

• Carbohydrates: 31g

• Dietary Fiber: 3g

• Fat: 0.5g

• Saturated Fat: 0g

• Sodium: 1mg

• Potassium: 320mg

• Phosphorus: 20mg

Pineapple Coconut Delight

A tropical and refreshing dessert that combines the sweetness of pineapple with the creamy texture of coconut milk. Prep Time: 5 minutes

Cooking Time: 0 minutes

Serving Size: 1 cup

Ingredients:

• 1 cup pineapple chunks

• 1/2 cup light coconut milk

• 1 tablespoon honey (optional)

Instructions:

In a blender, combine pineapple chunks and light coconut milk. Blend until smooth. Add honey if desired for extra sweetness. Serve immediately or chill for 30 minutes before serving.

Nutritional Information (per cup):

• Calories: 130

• Protein: 1g

• Carbohydrates: 27g

• Dietary Fiber: 2g

• Fat: 3g

• Saturated Fat: 2.5g

• Sodium: 10mg

• Potassium: 250mg

• Phosphorus: 20mg

Peach Frozen Yogurt

A creamy and delicious frozen yogurt made with ripe peaches, perfect for a healthy and refreshing dessert.
Prep Time: 5 minutes
Cooking Time: 0 minutes
Serving Size: 1 cup

Ingredients:

• 2 ripe peaches, peeled and sliced

• 1 cup low-fat Greek yogurt

• 1 tablespoon honey

Instructions:

In a blender, combine peaches, Greek yogurt, and honey. Blend until smooth. Pour the mixture into a shallow container and freeze for at least 4 hours. Before serving, let the frozen yogurt sit at room temperature for 5 minutes to soften slightly.

Nutritional Information (per cup):

• Calories: 180

- Protein: 8g
- Carbohydrates: 34g
- Dietary Fiber: 3g
- Fat: 2g
- Saturated Fat: 1g
- Sodium: 50mg
- Potassium: 400mg
- Phosphorus: 150mg

Raspberry Oat Bars

A healthy and tasty treat made with oats and fresh raspberries, perfect for a snack or dessert.

Prep Time: 10 minutes
Cooking Time: 30 minutes
Serving Size: 1 cup

Ingredients:
- 1 cup rolled oats
- 1/4 cup whole wheat flour
- 1/4 cup honey
- 1/4 cup unsweetened applesauce
- 1 cup raspberries

Instructions:

Preheat the oven to 350°F (175°C). In a bowl, combine rolled oats, whole wheat flour, honey, and applesauce. Mix well. Press half of the oat mixture into the bottom of a baking dish. Spread raspberries evenly over the oat mixture. Top with the remaining oat mixture and press down gently. Bake for 30 minutes or until golden brown. Let cool before cutting into bars.

Nutritional Information (per cup):

- Calories: 200
- Protein: 4g
- Carbohydrates: 40g
- Dietary Fiber: 6g
- Fat: 3g
- Saturated Fat: 0.5g
- Sodium: 10mg
- Potassium: 200mg
- Phosphorus: 100mg

Banana Oat Cookies

A healthy and simple cookie recipe made with ripe bananas and oats, perfect for a sweet snack.

Prep Time: 5 minutes

Cooking Time: 15 minutes

Serving Size: 1 cup

Ingredients:

• 2 ripe bananas, mashed

• 1 cup rolled oats

• 1/4 cup raisins

• 1 teaspoon cinnamon

Instructions:

Preheat the oven to 350°F (175°C). In a bowl, combine mashed bananas, rolled oats, raisins, and cinnamon. Mix well. Drop spoonfuls of the mixture onto a baking sheet lined with parchment paper. Flatten each cookie slightly. Bake for 15 minutes or until golden brown. Let cool before serving.

Nutritional Information (per cup):

• Calories: 150

• Protein: 3g

• Carbohydrates: 33g

• Dietary Fiber: 4g

• Fat: 2g

• Saturated Fat: 0.5g

- Sodium: 1mg
- Potassium: 300mg
- Phosphorus: 80mg

Delicious Desserts without the Guilt

Chocolate Avocado Mousse

A creamy and indulgent mousse made with avocados and cocoa powder, providing a healthy twist on a classic dessert.

Prep Time: 10 minutes
Cooking Time: 0 minutes
Serving Size: 1 cup

Ingredients:
- 1 ripe avocado
- 2 tablespoons unsweetened cocoa powder
- 2 tablespoons honey
- 1/4 cup almond milk
- 1 teaspoon vanilla extract

Instructions:

Cut the avocado in half, remove the pit, and scoop the flesh into a blender. Add cocoa powder, honey, almond milk, and vanilla extract. Blend until smooth and creamy. Transfer to serving bowls and chill in the refrigerator for at least 30 minutes before serving.

Nutritional Information (per cup):
- Calories: 210
- Protein: 3g
- Carbohydrates: 29g
- Dietary Fiber: 9g
- Fat: 11g
- Saturated Fat: 2g
- Sodium: 50mg
- Potassium: 660mg
- Phosphorus: 80mg

Vanilla Chia Seed Pudding

A simple and nutritious dessert made with chia seeds and vanilla, perfect for a light and satisfying treat.

Prep Time: 5 minutes

Cooking Time: 0 minutes

Serving Size: 1 cup

Ingredients:

- 1/4 cup chia seeds
- 1 cup almond milk
- 1 tablespoon honey
- 1 teaspoon vanilla extract

Instructions:

In a bowl, combine chia seeds, almond milk, honey, and vanilla extract. Stir well to prevent clumping. Refrigerate for at least 4 hours or overnight until the mixture thickens. Serve chilled.

Nutritional Information (per cup):

- Calories: 200
- Protein: 5g
- Carbohydrates: 22g
- Dietary Fiber: 11g
- Fat: 11g
- Saturated Fat: 1g
- Sodium: 60mg

- Potassium: 290mg
- Phosphorus: 220mg

Berry Frozen Yogurt Bark

A refreshing and fruity dessert made with Greek yogurt and mixed berries, perfect for a guilt-free treat.

Prep Time: 10 minutes
Cooking Time: 0 minutes
Serving Size: 1 cup

Ingredients:
- 1 cup low-fat Greek yogurt
- 1/2 cup mixed berries (blueberries, strawberries, raspberries)
- 1 tablespoon honey
- 1 teaspoon vanilla extract

Instructions:
Line a baking sheet with parchment paper. In a bowl, mix Greek yogurt, honey, and vanilla extract. Spread the yogurt mixture evenly on the baking sheet. Sprinkle mixed berries on top. Freeze for at least 2 hours. Break into pieces before serving.

Nutritional Information (per cup):

• Calories: 130

• Protein: 10g

• Carbohydrates: 22g

• Dietary Fiber: 3g

• Fat: 1.5g

• Saturated Fat: 1g

• Sodium: 50mg

• Potassium: 300mg

• Phosphorus: 150mg

Mango Coconut Pudding

A creamy and tropical dessert made with fresh mangoes and coconut milk, perfect for a light and refreshing treat.

Prep Time: 10 minutes
Cooking Time: 0 minutes
Serving Size: 1 cup

Ingredients:

• 1 ripe mango, peeled and diced

• 1/2 cup light coconut milk

- 1 tablespoon honey
- 1 teaspoon lime juice

Instructions:

In a blender, combine mango, coconut milk, honey, and lime juice. Blend until smooth. Pour the mixture into serving bowls and chill in the refrigerator for at least 1 hour before serving.

Nutritional Information (per cup):
- Calories: 180
- Protein: 2g
- Carbohydrates: 35g
- Dietary Fiber: 3g
- Fat: 4g
- Saturated Fat: 3.5g
- Sodium: 10mg
- Potassium: 300mg
- Phosphorus: 30mg

Baked Cinnamon Apples

A warm and comforting dessert made with baked apples and cinnamon, perfect for a healthy and delicious treat.

Prep Time: 10 minutes

Cooking Time: 20 minutes

Serving Size: 1 cup

Ingredients:

- 2 apples, cored and sliced
- 1 teaspoon ground cinnamon
- 1 tablespoon honey

Instructions:

Preheat the oven to 350°F (175°C). In a bowl, toss apple slices with cinnamon and honey. Arrange the apple slices in a baking dish. Bake for 20 minutes or until tender. Serve warm.

Nutritional Information (per cup):

- Calories: 150
- Protein: 0.5g
- Carbohydrates: 40g
- Dietary Fiber: 6g
- Fat: 0.5g
- Saturated Fat: 0g
- Sodium: 0mg
- Potassium: 260mg
- Phosphorus: 20mg

Orange Sorbet

A refreshing and citrusy dessert made with fresh oranges, perfect for a light and guilt-free treat.

Prep Time: 10 minutes
Cooking Time: 0 minutes
Serving Size: 1 cup

Ingredients:
- 3 large oranges, juiced
- 1 tablespoon honey
- 1 teaspoon lemon juice

Instructions:
In a blender, combine orange juice, honey, and lemon juice. Blend until well mixed. Pour the mixture into a shallow container and freeze for at least 4 hours. Stir occasionally to break up ice crystals. Serve as a scoopable sorbet.

Nutritional Information (per cup):
- Calories: 100
- Protein: 1g
- Carbohydrates: 25g

- Dietary Fiber: 2g
- Fat: 0g
- Saturated Fat: 0g
- Sodium: 1mg
- Potassium: 350mg
- Phosphorus: 30mg

Banana Oat Muffins

A healthy and delicious muffin made with ripe bananas and oats, perfect for a sweet and satisfying dessert.

Prep Time: 10 minutes
Cooking Time: 20 minutes
Serving Size: 1 cup

Ingredients:
- 2 ripe bananas, mashed
- 1 cup rolled oats
- 1/4 cup honey
- 1 teaspoon baking powder
- 1 teaspoon vanilla extract

Instructions:

Preheat the oven to 350°F (175°C). In a bowl, mix mashed bananas, rolled oats, honey, baking powder, and vanilla extract. Pour the batter into a muffin tin lined with paper cups. Bake for 20 minutes or until golden brown. Let cool before serving.

Nutritional Information (per cup):

- Calories: 150
- Protein: 3g
- Carbohydrates: 35g
- Dietary Fiber: 4g
- Fat: 1g
- Saturated Fat: 0g
- Sodium: 50mg
- Potassium: 300mg
- Phosphorus: 80mg

Coconut Rice Pudding

A creamy and delightful pudding made with rice and coconut milk, providing a tropical twist to a classic dessert.

Prep Time: 10 minutes

Cooking Time: 25 minutes

Serving Size: 1 cup

Ingredients:

- 1/2 cup cooked white rice
- 1 cup light coconut milk
- 1 tablespoon honey
- 1 teaspoon vanilla extract

Instructions:

In a saucepan, combine cooked rice, coconut milk, honey, and vanilla extract. Cook over medium heat, stirring occasionally, until the mixture thickens, about 20-25 minutes. Serve warm or chilled.

Nutritional Information (per cup):

- Calories: 180
- Protein: 3g
- Carbohydrates: 30g
- Dietary Fiber: 1g
- Fat: 6g
- Saturated Fat: 5g
- Sodium: 20mg

- Potassium: 150mg

- Phosphorus: 40mg

Lemon Yogurt Cake

A light and zesty cake made with yogurt and lemon, perfect for a refreshing and guilt-free dessert.

Prep Time: 10 minutes
Cooking Time: 25 minutes
Serving Size: 1 cup

Ingredients:
- 1 cup low-fat Greek yogurt
- 1/2 cup whole wheat flour
- 1/4 cup honey
- 1 egg
- 1 teaspoon baking powder
- 1 teaspoon lemon zest

Instructions:
Preheat the oven to 350°F (175°C). In a bowl, mix Greek yogurt, whole wheat flour, honey, egg, baking powder, and lemon zest. Pour the batter into a greased baking

dish. Bake for 25 minutes or until a toothpick inserted in the center comes out clean. Let cool before serving.

Nutritional Information (per cup):

• Calories: 200

• Protein: 8g

• Carbohydrates: 30g

• Dietary Fiber: 2g

• Fat: 5g

• Saturated Fat: 1.5g

• Sodium: 60mg

• Potassium: 200mg

• Phosphorus: 100mg

Peach Cobbler

A healthy and delicious cobbler made with fresh peaches and a light, whole grain topping.

Prep Time: 10 minutes
Cooking Time: 20 minutes
Serving Size: 1 cup

Ingredients:

• 2 ripe peaches, sliced

- 1/4 cup whole wheat flour
- 1/4 cup rolled oats
- 2 tablespoons honey
- 1 teaspoon cinnamon
- 1 tablespoon coconut oil, melted

Instructions:

Preheat the oven to 350°F (175°C). In a baking dish, arrange sliced peaches. In a bowl, mix whole wheat flour, rolled oats, honey, cinnamon, and melted coconut oil. Sprinkle the mixture over the peaches. Bake for 20 minutes or until the topping is golden brown. Serve warm.

Nutritional Information (per cup):

- Calories: 160
- Protein: 3g
- Carbohydrates: 33g
- Dietary Fiber: 4g
- Fat: 3g
- Saturated Fat: 2g
- Sodium: 5mg
- Potassium: 300mg
- Phosphorus: 70mg

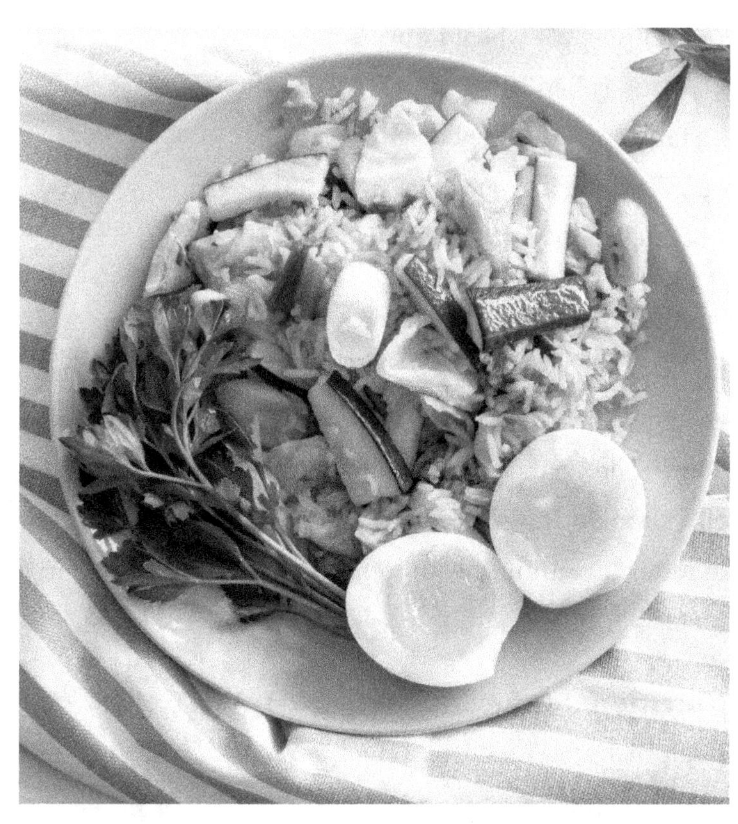

CHAPTER 9: 90-DAY MEAL PLAN

DAYS	BREAKFAST	LUNCH	DINNER
1.	Quinoa with apples and cinnamon	Quinoa salad with vegetables	Lemon herb baked chicken
2.	Blueberry Banana Smoothie	Lentil Vegetable Soup	Baked Salmon with Asparagus
3.	Vanilla Chia Seed Pudding	Turkey and Avocado Wrap	Stir-Fried Tofu with Vegetables
4.	Overnight Oats with Almonds	Chickpea Salad	Grilled Shrimp with

			Quinoa
5.	Greek Yogurt with Honey and Berries	Tomato and Cucumber Sandwich	Vegetable Stir-Fry with Brown Rice
6.	Scrambled EggWhites with Spinach	Chicken and Hummus Wrap Lemon	Garlic Chicken with Broccoli
7.	Avocado Toast with Tomatoes	Lentil and Spinach Salad	Grilled Tilapia with

			Green Beans
8.	Smoothie Bowl with Mixed Fruits	Black Bean Soup	Baked Chicken with Sweet Potatoes
9.	Quinoa Breakfast Bowl with Berries	Tuna Salad	Turkey Meatballs with Zucchini Noodles
10.	Apple Cinnamon Oatmeal	Grilled Chicken Salad	Shrimp and Vegetable Skewers

11.	Mango Smoothie	Quinoa and Black Bean Bowl	Lemon Baked Cod with Spinach
12.	Banana Oat Pancakes	Turkey and Cheese Sandwich	Grilled Veggie Kebabs
13.	Greek Yogurt Parfait	Lentil and Quinoa Salad	Baked Chicken with Brussels Sprouts
14.	Spinach and Mushroom Omelet	Chickpea and Avocado	Grilled Salmon with

		Wrap	Quinoa
15.	Chia Seed Pudding with Mango	Tomato Basil Soup	Tofu Stir-Fry with Brown Rice
16.	Berry Smoothie	Quinoa Salad with Kale	Baked Tilapia with Vegetables
17.	Overnight Oats with Chia Seeds	Turkey Lettuce Wraps	Lemon Garlic Shrimp with Asparagus
18.	Apple Walnut Breakfast Bowl	Chickpea and	Grilled Chicken

		Cucumber Salad	with Broccoli
19.	Spinach and Banana Smoothie	Tuna Salad Lettuce Wraps	Stir-Fried Tofu with Mixed Veggies
20.	Greek Yogurt with Nuts and Berries	Quinoa and Black Bean Salad	Baked Salmon with Spinach
21.	Scrambled Eggs with Tomatoes	Grilled Vegetable Sandwich	Lemon Herb Chicken with Sweet Potatoes

22.	Avocado and	Lentil Soup	Grilled

	Egg Toast		Shrimp with Quinoa
23.	Smoothie Bowl with Almond Butter	Turkey and Avocado Salad	Baked Cod with Green Beans
24.	Chia Seed Pudding with Berries	Quinoa and Chickpea Salad	Lemon Garlic Chicken with Brussels Sprouts
25.	Apple Cinnamon Overnight Oats	Spinach and Feta Wrap	Grilled Salmon with Brown Rice

26.	Mango Banana Smoothie	Black Bean and Corn Salad	Baked Chicken with Asparagus
27.	Greek Yogurt Parfait with Granola	Tomato Basil Wrap	Stir-Fried Tofu with Broccoli
28.	Scrambled Eggs with Spinach	Quinoa and Vegetable Bowl	Lemon Baked Tilapia with Vegetables
29.	Berry Banana Smoothie	Turkey and Cheese Lettuce Wrap	Grilled Shrimp with Green Beans

30.	Chia Seed Pudding with Coconut	Lentil and Avocado Salad	Baked Chicken with Sweet Potatoes
31.	Apple Walnut Oatmeal	Quinoa Salad with Kale	Grilled Salmon with Spinach
32.	Smoothie Bowl with Mixed Berries	Chickpea and Tomato Salad	Stir-Fried Tofu with Brown Rice
33.	Greek Yogurt with Honey and Nuts	Tuna Salad with Avocado	Lemon Garlic Chicken with Broccoli

34.	Spinach and Mushroom Omelet	Quinoa and Black Bean Wrap	Baked Cod with Vegetables
35.	Avocado and Tomato Toast	Lentil and Spinach Wrap	Grilled Shrimp with Quinoa
36.	Banana Almond Smoothie	Turkey and Cheese Salad	Baked Chicken with Brussels Sprouts
37.	Chia Seed Pudding with Mango	Quinoa and Chickpea Bowl	Grilled Salmon with

			Asparagus
38.	Berry Oatmeal	Tomato Basil Salad	Stir-Fried Tofu with Green Beans
39.	Greek Yogurt with Mixed Fruits	Grilled Chicken Wrap	Lemon Garlic Shrimp with Brown Rice
40.	Spinach and Egg White Scramble	Black Bean and Corn Wrap	Baked Tilapia with Vegetables
41.	Avocado	Quinoa	Grilled

	Banana Smoothie	Salad with Spinach	Chicken with Sweet Potatoes
42.	Chia Seed Pudding with Blueberries	Chickpea and Avocado Wrap	Baked Salmon with Quinoa
43.	Apple Cinnamon Oatmeal	Tomato Basil Wrap	Stir-Fried Tofu with Broccoli
44.	Mango Smoothie	Turkey and Cheese Lettuce Wrap	Lemon Baked Cod with Spinach
45.	Greek Yogurt Parfait	Quinoa and Vegetable	Grilled Shrimp

		Salad	with Green Beans
46.	Scrambled Eggs with Tomatoes	Lentil and Avocado Salad	Baked Chicken with Asparagus
47.	Berry Smoothie Bowl	Quinoa Salad with Kale	Stir-Fried Tofu with Brown Rice
48.	Greek Yogurt with Granola	Chickpea and Tomato Wrap	Lemon Garlic Chicken with Broccoli
49.	Spinach and Mushroom	Tuna Salad with	Baked Cod with

	Omelet	Avocado	Vegetables
50.	Avocado and Egg Toast	Quinoa and Black Bean Wrap	Grilled Shrimp with Sweet Potatoes
51.	Smoothie Bowl with Almond Butter	Lentil and Spinach Wrap	Baked Chicken with Brussels Sprouts
52.	Chia Seed Pudding with Berries	Turkey and Cheese Salad	Grilled Salmon with Asparagus
53.	Apple Cinnamon	Quinoa and Chickpea	Stir-Fried Tofu with

	Overnight Oats	Bowl	Green Beans
54.	Mango Banana Smoothie	Black Bean and Corn Wrap	Lemon Garlic Shrimp with Brown Rice
55.	Greek Yogurt Parfait with Granola	Quinoa Salad with Spinach	Baked Tilapia with Vegetables
56.	Scrambled Eggs with Spinach	Chickpea and Avocado Salad	Grilled Chicken with Sweet Potatoes
57.	Berry Banana Smoothie	Tuna Salad with Avocado	Baked Salmon with

			Quinoa
58.	Chia Seed Pudding with Coconut	Quinoa and Vegetable Wrap	Stir-Fried Tofu with Broccoli
59.	Apple Walnut Oatmeal	Lentil and Avocado Wrap	Lemon Baked Cod with Spinach
60.	Smoothie Bowl with Mixed Berries	Turkey and Cheese Lettuce Wrap	Grilled Shrimp with Green Beans
61.	Greek Yogurt with Honey and Nuts	Quinoa Salad with Kale	Baked Chicken with Asparagus

62.	Spinach and Mushroom Omelet	Chickpea and Tomato Salad	Stir-Fried Tofu with Brown Rice
63.	Avocado and Tomato Toast	Tuna Salad with Avocado	Lemon Garlic Chicken with Broccoli
64.	Banana Almond Smoothie	Quinoa and Black Bean Wrap	Baked Cod with Vegetables
65.	Chia Seed Pudding with Mango	Lentil and Spinach Wrap	Grilled Shrimp with Sweet Potatoes
66.	Berry	Turkey and	Baked

	Oatmeal	Cheese Salad	Chicken with Brussels Sprouts
67.	Greek Yogurt with Mixed Fruits	Quinoa and Chickpea Bowl	Grilled Salmon with Asparagus
68.	Spinach and Egg White Scramble	Black Bean and Corn Wrap	Stir-Fried Tofu with Green Beans
69.	Avocado Banana Smoothie	Quinoa Salad with Spinach	Lemon Garlic Shrimp with Brown

			Rice
70.	Chia Seed Pudding with Blueberries	Chickpea and Avocado Wrap	Baked Tilapia with Vegetables
71.	Apple Cinnamon Oatmeal	Tomato Basil Wrap	Grilled Chicken with Sweet Potatoes
72.	Mango Smoothie	Turkey and Cheese Lettuce Wrap	Baked Salmon with Quinoa
73.	Greek Yogurt Parfait	Quinoa and Vegetable Salad	Stir-Fried Tofu with Broccoli

74.	Scrambled Eggs with Tomatoes	Lentil and Avocado Salad	Lemon Baked Cod with Spinach
75.	Berry Smoothie Bowl	Quinoa Salad with Kale	Grilled Shrimp with Green Beans
76.	Greek Yogurt with Granola	Chickpea and Tomato Wrap	Baked Chicken with Asparagus
77.	Spinach and Mushroom Omelet	Tuna Salad with Avocado	Stir-Fried Tofu with Brown Rice
78.	Avocado and	Quinoa and	Lemon

	Egg Toast	Black Bean Wrap	Garlic Chicken with Broccoli
79.	Smoothie Bowl with Almond Butter	Lentil and Spinach Wrap	Baked Cod with Vegetables
80.	Chia Seed Pudding with Berries	Turkey and Cheese Salad	Grilled Shrimp with Sweet Potatoes
81.	Apple Cinnamon Overnight	Quinoa and Chickpea Bowl	Baked Chicken with

	Oats		Brussels Sprouts
82.	Mango Banana Smoothie	Black Bean and Corn Wrap	Grilled Salmon with Asparagus
83.	Greek Yogurt Parfait with Granola	Quinoa Salad with Spinach	Stir-Fried Tofu with Green Beans
84.	Scrambled Eggs with Spinach	Chickpea and Avocado Salad	Lemon Garlic Shrimp with Brown

			Rice
85.	Berry Banana Smoothie	Tuna Salad with Avocado	Baked Tilapia with Vegetables
86.	Chia Seed Pudding with Coconut	Quinoa and Vegetable Wrap	Grilled Chicken with Sweet Potatoes
87.	Apple Walnut Oatmeal	Lentil and Avocado Wrap	Baked Salmon with Quinoa
88.	Smoothie Bowl with	Turkey and Cheese	Stir-Fried Tofu with

	Mixed Berries	Lettuce Wrap	Broccoli

89.	Greek Yogurt with Honey and Nuts	Quinoa Salad with Kale	Lemon Baked Cod with Spinach
90.	Spinach and Mushroom Omelet	Chickpea and Tomato Salad	Grilled Shrimp with Green Beans

This plan uses a variety of recipes regularly to keep things interesting and ensure a healthy diet. Each meal is low in fat, uses ingredients that are easy to find and is affordable. Have fun on your way to eating better!

CHAPTER 10: EXPERT TIPS FOR POST-SURGERY RECOVERY

Expert Tips for Post-Surgery Recovery

Recovery from gallbladder surgery can be a difficult process that necessitates dietary and lifestyle changes to manage digestive health and ensure a quick recovery. As a specialist nutritionist, I will give far-reaching direction on overseeing stomach-related well-being, ways to remain focused on your healing, and laying out long-haul good dieting propensities. These methods are intended to support your overall health and assist you in effectively navigating life after surgery.

Managing Digestive Health

After the gallbladder medical procedure, your stomach-related framework needs time to adjust to the shortfall of the gallbladder, which assumes a pivotal part in bile capacity and fat processing. To oversee stomach-related well-being, it is crucial to roll out dietary improvements that advance stomach-related effectiveness and limit uneasiness. First, center around integrating low-fat food varieties into your eating routine. The gallbladder stores bile, which helps separate fats. Without it, your body will find it more testing to process high-fat food varieties, possibly prompting loose bowels, swelling, and stomach torment. Include plenty of fruits, vegetables, whole grains, and legumes, as well as lean proteins like fish, chicken, and turkey. Not only are these foods low in fat, but they also contain a lot of fiber, which helps with digestion and prevents constipation. Also, consider eating more modest, successive meals over the day rather than three enormous ones. This method makes it possible to absorb nutrients more effectively while avoiding overtaxing your digestive system. More modest dinners likewise lessen the probability of encountering postprandial distress. Another important aspect of managing digestive health is staying hydrated. Throughout the day, drinking a lot of water aids in maintaining regular bowel movements and supports overall digestive function. Drink at least eight glasses of water daily, and steer clear of drinks high in sugar and caffeine, which can aggravate digestive issues. Introduce food varieties that advance stomach well-being, like probiotics and prebiotics. Probiotics, tracked down in yogurt, kefir, and matured food varieties, contain useful microorganisms that help a solid stomach microbiome. These good bacteria are fed by prebiotics, which are found in foods like garlic, onions, and bananas. This makes them more effective.

Last but not least, avoid foods that can make your stomach hurt. Spicy foods, high-fiber foods like beans and cruciferous vegetables, and carbonated beverages are all common culprits. You can make your recovery process go more smoothly by keeping a food diary, which can help you identify and eliminate these triggers from your diet.

Tips for Staying on Track

Discipline, support, and practical strategies are all required to continue your recovery after gallbladder surgery. The following expert advice will assist you in maintaining your progress and completing a successful recovery. First and foremost, establish objectives and expectations that are attainable. Recognize that recovery is a gradual process and that dietary changes may take some time to show results. Keep being patient with yourself as you adjust to new eating habits and changes in your lifestyle, and remember to celebrate the little victories along the way. Utilize the assistance of healthcare professionals, such as a registered dietitian or nutritionist, who can offer individualized guidance tailored to your particular requirements and circumstances. You can get expert advice on how to deal with any difficulties you face during your recovery from regular consultations, which can assist you in remaining accountable. Include meal preparation and planning into your daily routine. Plan your meals for the coming week with a focus on well-balanced, low-fat options that are good for digestion. Planning feasts ahead of time can assist you with staying away from the allurement of undesirable decisions and guarantee you have nutritious choices promptly accessible. Practice careful eating by focusing on your body's yearning and completion signals. Eat gradually and relish each chomp, permitting your stomach-related framework time to productively handle food. This approach can assist with forestalling indulging and lessen the probability of encountering stomach-related uneasiness. Maintain your physical activity and incorporate it into your daily routine regularly. Exercise has been shown to improve digestion, mood, and overall health. On most days of the week, aim for at least 30 minutes of moderate exercise, such as walking, swimming, or cycling. Make certain to counsel your medical care supplier before beginning any new activity routine to guarantee it is right for your post-medical procedure recuperation. Keep a positive outlook and remain roused by helping yourself to remember the drawn-out advantages of your dietary and way of life changes. Keep a journal to record your progress reflect on your journey and visualize your goals. Encircle yourself with a strong organization of loved ones who can offer support and help depending on the situation.

Long-Term Healthy Eating Habits

Laying out long-haul good dieting propensities is fundamental for keeping up with stomach-related well-being and by and large prosperity after a gallbladder medical procedure. These propensities won't just help your recovery but additionally add to a better way of life in the years to come. Center around a reasonable eating routine that incorporates different supplements and tasty food sources. Include a lot of fruits and vegetables, whole grains, lean proteins, and healthy fats like olive oil, nuts, and avocados. This method guarantees that you get all of the necessary vitamins, minerals, and nutrients your body needs to work at its best. Limit your admission of handled and high-fat food sources, which can be trying for your stomach-related framework. Choose whole, unprocessed foods because they are easier to digest and contain more nutrients. Choose cooking methods that minimize added fats, such as baking, steaming, and grilling, and carefully read food labels to avoid hidden fats and additives. To effectively manage your weight and prevent overeating, practice portion control. Utilize more modest plates and bowls to assist with managing segment estimates, and pay attention to your body's appetite and completion signals.

Find healthy ways to cope with emotions, such as engaging in physical activity or practicing mindfulness techniques, and avoid eating out of boredom or stress. Drink plenty of water throughout the day to keep hydrated. Appropriate hydration upholds absorption, manages internal heat levels, and keeps your skin sound. Avoid beverages with caffeine or sugar because they can dehydrate you and exacerbate digestive issues. By including probiotics and prebiotics in your diet, you can maintain your focus on gut health. These helpful parts support a solid stomach microbiome, which is essential for proficient processing and general well-being. You can easily incorporate probiotic-rich foods like yogurt, kefir, sauerkraut, and kimchi into your diet by experimenting with a variety of them.

At last, teach yourself about sustenance and remain informed about the most recent dietary suggestions. You can take charge of your health and make well-informed choices with the knowledge you have. You might want to consider joining an online community or support group where you can learn from others who have been through similar experiences and share your own. You can ensure a successful post-surgery recovery and lead a healthier, more satisfying life by practicing these expert suggestions for managing digestive health, staying on track with your recovery, and developing long-term healthy eating habits. Keep in mind, that the excursion to ideal well-being is a ceaseless cycle, and rolling out

feasible improvements will yield enduring advantages
for your general prosperity.

CHAPTER 11: MAINTAINING METABOLIC BALANCE

Maintaining Metabolic Balance

Maintaining metabolic equilibrium after a gallbladder medical procedure is vital for well-being and prosperity. The removal of the gallbladder necessitates changes in diet and lifestyle to ensure that metabolic processes continue to run smoothly because the gallbladder plays a significant role in fat digestion. This part will dive into the job of digestion post-medical procedure, distinguish food varieties that support digestion, and give exercise and way-of-life tips to assist you with keeping a fair metabolic rate.

The Role of Metabolism Post-Surgery

Digestion is the arrangement of life-supporting substance responses in the body, including those that convert food into energy, construct and fix tissues, and dispense with byproducts. As the body adjusts to the gallbladder's absence after surgery, several changes occur. Understanding these progressions is fundamental to keeping up with metabolic equilibrium. After gallbladder evacuation, the liver keeps on delivering bile, however, it is delivered straightforwardly into the small digestive system as opposed to being put away and amassed in the gallbladder. This consistent, less focused bile stream can make fat processing less effective, which might prompt side effects like runs, swelling, and gas if the eating regimen isn't changed as needed. Therefore, to support metabolic equilibrium and prevent these issues, it is essential to control fat intake. During recovery and surgery, the body's overall metabolic rate may also be affected. Alterations in diet and reduced physical activity can slow metabolism during the recovery phase. It's vital to progressively introduce actual work and a decent eating routine to reestablish and keep up with the metabolic rate. A fair eating routine that incorporates the right extent of macronutrients (sugars, proteins, and fats) is crucial. Lean proteins, complex carbohydrates, and healthy fats can help ensure that the body has the fuel it needs to continue metabolic processes after surgery. Hydration likewise assumes a basic part in digestion, as water is important for different metabolic responses, including the breakdown of food and the disposal of side effects.

Furthermore, metabolic health depends on micronutrients like vitamins and minerals. Because they aid in the conversion of food into energy, vitamins like the B-complex (B6, B12, and folic acid) are particularly important. Muscle function and energy production are supported by minerals like iron and magnesium.

Foods that Boost Metabolism

Consuming certain foods can raise your metabolic rate, which helps you use energy more effectively and control your weight. After surgery, eating these foods can help you keep your metabolism in check. Foods high in protein have the greatest effect on increasing metabolism. The energy required to digest, absorb, and process nutrients is known as the thermic effect of food (TEF). Protein has a higher TEF compared to fats and starches, meaning the body consumes more calories handling protein. Lean meats, poultry, fish, eggs, dairy items, vegetables, and soy items are fantastic wellsprings of protein that can assist with supporting digestion. Another group of foods that can speed up metabolism is whole grains. Not all refined grains, entire grains contain all pieces of the grain, including the wheat, microorganism, and endosperm. Because of this, they contain more nutrients and fiber, both of which require more energy to digest. Oats, brown rice, quinoa, and whole wheat products are examples of whole grains. Consuming hot foods, especially those that contain capsaicin, can also raise metabolic rates. It has been demonstrated that chili peppers' capsaicin boosts calorie burning and fat oxidation. Adding moderate measures of hot food sources to your eating regimen can give your digestion an impermanent lift. Coffee and green tea are well-known beverages for their ability to speed up metabolism. Catechins are antioxidants that can boost fat burning and are found in green tea. Caffeine, which can raise metabolic rate and enhance physical performance, is found in coffee. However, to avoid potential side effects like a faster heart rate or discomfort in the digestive tract, it is essential to consume these beverages in moderation.

Integrating leafy foods into your eating routine is fundamental for general well-being and digestion. Food sources like apples, berries, spinach, and broccoli are high in fiber, nutrients, and cancer-prevention agents, which support metabolic well-being. Fiber-rich food sources likewise help in processing and controlling glucose levels, adding to fair digestion. Solid fats, albeit required in more modest sums post-medical procedure, are additionally significant. Avocados, olive oil, nuts, and seeds are all good sources of healthy fats. Without the negative effects of saturated and trans fats, these fats help cells function and generate energy.

Exercise and Lifestyle Tips

Actual work and way-of-life decisions assume a critical part in keeping up with metabolic equilibrium. One of the best ways to improve overall health and speed up metabolism is to exercise regularly. Walking, jogging, swimming, cycling, and other aerobic activities raise heart rate and help burn calories. A significant increase in metabolic rate can be achieved by including at least 150 minutes of moderate aerobic activity or 75 minutes of vigorous activity each week. It is best to begin with light exercises like walking for people recovering from surgery and gradually increase the intensity. Strength preparation is one more significant part of keeping up with metabolic equilibrium. Building bulk through practices like powerlifting, obstruction band exercises, or bodyweight works out, (for example, push-ups and squats) can increment resting metabolic rate. Increasing muscle mass helps maintain a higher metabolic rate because muscle tissue burns more calories at rest than fat tissue. Incorporating more physical activity into daily routines can help support metabolic balance in addition to structured exercise. Straightforward changes like using the stairwell rather than the lift, strolling or trekking for little excursions, and standing or moving around during breaks can add to general calorie consumption.

Additionally, metabolic health depends on getting enough sleep. Sleep deprivation can alter hormones that control hunger and metabolism, resulting in weight gain and a slower metabolic rate. To support metabolism and overall health, aim for 7-9 hours of quality sleep each night. Another crucial aspect of maintaining metabolic equilibrium is stress management. Persistent pressure can prompt hormonal uneven characters that adversely influence digestion.

Engaging in hobbies, mindfulness meditation, yoga, and deep breathing exercises can support metabolic health and reduce stress. At long last, remaining hydrated is fundamental for metabolic cycles. Water is essential for assimilation, supplement retention, and waste end. Your body will be able to carry out these tasks in an effective manner if you consume enough water throughout the day. Drink at least 8 cups (64 ounces) of water daily as a general rule, but each person's requirements may vary. You can support overall well-being and maintain metabolic equilibrium by understanding the role of metabolism after surgery, incorporating foods that boost metabolism, and adopting healthy exercise and lifestyle habits. These techniques will assist you with exploring the post-medical procedure time frame successfully and advance long-haul well-being and imperativeness.

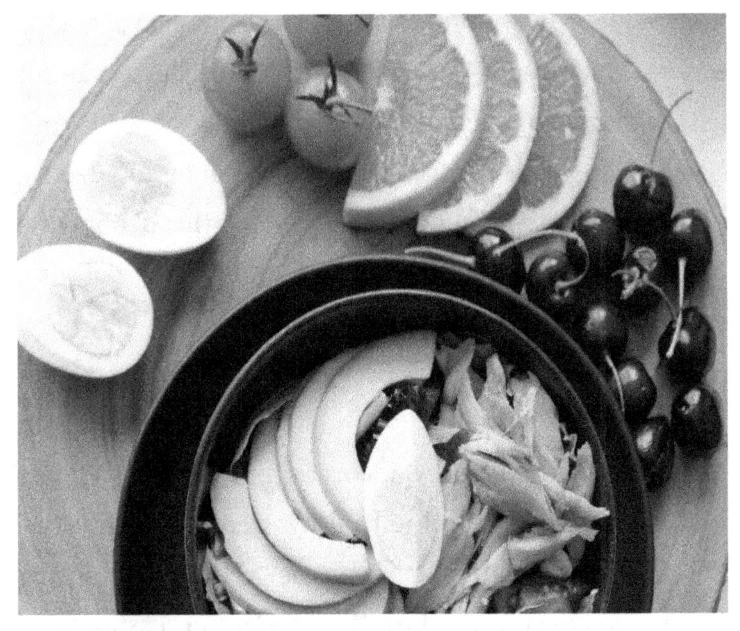

CHAPTER 12: PERSONAL STORIES AND TESTIMONIALS

Personal Stories and Testimonials

Each person's journey through gallbladder surgery and recovery is completely individual. This part unites genuine encounters, tips, and counsel from other people who have strolled this way, and inspirational examples of overcoming adversity to move and guide you. As you begin your journey, it can be helpful to gain valuable insights and encouragement from those who have overcome similar obstacles.

Real-Life Experiences

Experiences from real people give a sense of the many difficulties and successes that people who have had gallbladder surgery face. The initial adjustment to dietary changes is a recurring theme. A lot of people say that the body adjusts to not having the gallbladder for the first few weeks after surgery, which can be especially hard. For instance, Sarah, a 45-year-old teacher, talked about how she struggled with digestive issues and learned to control her diet over time. She at first confronted swelling and uneasiness yet tracked down alleviation by consolidating more modest, more incessant dinners and keeping away from high-fat food sources. During the recovery process, John, a 50-year-old accountant, stressed the significance of patience. He gained weight as a result of fatigue and a slower metabolism. As his energy levels improved, John emphasized the importance of incorporating moderate physical activity and gradually increasing intensity. His experience highlights that recuperation is certainly not a direct cycle, and it's fundamental to pay attention to your body and progress at an agreeable speed. Maria, a nurse in her 30s, had another real-world experience in that she had difficulty maintaining a healthy diet. She tried several foods and found that vegetables and whole grains, which are high in fiber, made her feel fuller and helped her digest food better. The trial-and-error nature of post-surgery diet adjustments and the significance of individual approaches are exemplified by Maria's story. These genuine encounters highlight that while the excursion might be testing, it is likewise sensible with the right procedures and a positive outlook. The sharing of individual experiences contributes to the development of a supportive community in which others can find comfort and direction.

Tips and Advice from Others

For navigating the recovery process, the collective wisdom of those who have undergone gallbladder surgery is invaluable. One of the most often referenced suggestions is to focus on a fair eating routine. Starting with bland, easy-to-digest foods and gradually introducing more complex meals is the advice of many. A common recommendation is to avoid foods high in fat and fried, as these can aggravate digestive issues. Another important aspect that is frequently emphasized is portion control. To avoid overtaxing the digestive system and minimize discomfort, eat smaller meals more regularly. Kelly, a mother of 42, suggests keeping a food diary to monitor what you eat and how it affects your body. This training can assist with distinguishing triggers and designing your eating routine according to your particular requirements. Remaining hydrated is a key tip shared by a few people. Drinking enough water helps digestion and keeps the metabolism in check.

Including herbal teas like ginger or peppermint tea can help with nausea and bloating by soothing the digestive system. It is generally recommended to incorporate moderate physical activity into lifestyle changes. Walking has many advantages, including low impact and adaptability to your fitness level.

Not only does exercise increase metabolism, but it also improves well-being and energy levels overall. Starting with short daily walks and gradually increasing their duration and intensity is the advice of many people. Throughout the recovery process, support networks are essential. Joining support gatherings, either face to face or on the web, can give a feeling of the local area and deal with viable exhortation. Sharing encounters and hearing from other people who have confronted comparable difficulties can be relieving and propelling. A common theme is to listen to your body and be patient with yourself. Recuperation takes time, and it's essential to recognize and regard your body's requirements. Frustration can result from rushing the process or comparing your progress to that of others. The path to recovery that each person takes is different, and if you treat yourself with compassion, you can make the process go more smoothly and make it more enjoyable.

Motivational Success Stories

Success stories show that it is possible to live a happy and healthy life after surgery, which is a powerful motivator. These accounts focus on people who have not only recovered but also thrived, embracing new lifestyles and achieving health objectives. Mark, a retired 60-year-old who underwent gallbladder surgery, is one example of such a story. At first, Mark had serious digestive issues and gained weight, but he stuck with a low-fat, high-fiber diet and regular exercise. He reported feeling more energetic and healthier than in years as he lost 30 pounds over time. Imprint's journey features the potential for positive change and the significance of diligence and devotion. Lila, a 35-year-old fitness fanatic, used her recovery to change her diet and exercise routine. She put a strong emphasis on including foods high in nutrients like vegetables, whole grains, and lean proteins. Lila likewise embraced yoga and pilates, which assisted her with recapturing strength and adaptability. Her story demonstrates that recovery can serve as a springboard for adopting a healthier way of life and achieving new fitness milestones. Emily, a student who was 28 years old, had trouble juggling her studies and recovery. She battled with pressure and uneasiness, which impacted her stomach-related well-being. Emily found solace in mindfulness practices like deep breathing exercises and meditation. These practices further developed her psychological prosperity as well as decidedly affected her processing. Emily's story features the interconnectedness of mental and actual well-being and the advantages of comprehensive methodologies. Tom, a 55-year-old businessman, is another inspiring story about how he initially felt overwhelmed by dietary restrictions. He decided to broaden his culinary horizons and began cooking as a hobby. Tom developed a passion for healthy cooking through his experiments with various low-fat recipes. His journey exemplifies how recovery can improve the overall quality of life by opening doors to new hobbies and interests. These inspiring success stories demonstrate that, despite the ups and downs of the recovery path, there are opportunities for growth and positive transformation. Each story shows the human spirit's tenacity and the possibility of recovering from surgery to lead a healthier, more satisfying life.

In conclusion, individuals navigating post-surgery recovery can find information, encouragement, and support in personal stories and testimonials. Genuine encounters offer pragmatic experiences, tips, and encouragements from others featuring powerful techniques and inspirational examples of overcoming adversity that help us remember the opportunities for positive change. By associating with these accounts, people can track down solace, direction, and inspiration on their journey to recovery and prosperity.

Resources

Having the right resources at your disposal can significantly ease the process of recovering from surgery and maintaining a healthy lifestyle. This section gives a thorough manual for valuable sites and applications, suggested perusing, and care groups and networks. To assist you in achieving your health objectives and effectively managing your condition, these resources are intended to provide direction, support, and useful information.

Useful Websites and Apps

The web is a gold mine of data, and a few sites and applications can assist you with dealing with your post-medical procedure recuperation and long-haul well-being. For dependable clinical counsel and data, sites like Mayo Center and WebMD offer broad assets on gallbladder wellbeing, dietary suggestions, and recuperation tips. To help you along your journey, these websites offer articles that have been reviewed by medical professionals, testimonials from patients, and expert advice. Websites devoted to nutrition, such as Nutrition.gov and the Academy of Nutrition and Dietetics, provide useful information regarding healthy eating, meal planning, and balanced diets. In addition to low-fat recipes and nutritional guidelines, these websites offer resources for creating individualized meal plans that are tailored to your particular dietary requirements. MyFitnessPal is a popular option for tracking your diet and exercise for those who prefer mobile apps. You can log your meals, keep track of how many calories you consume, and keep track of how much you move with this app. It also has a large food database, making it easier to find nutritional information and stay on track with your dietary objectives. Another helpful application is Yummly, which gives customized recipe suggestions given your dietary inclinations and limitations. Yummly's extensive recipe collection includes meals that are good for the gallbladder and low in fat, making it easier to find healthy and delicious meals that meet your needs. Moreover, the application Noom offers an extensive way to deal with weight the board and sound living. It joins customized instructing, dinner following, and instructive assets to assist you with making maintainable way-of-life changes. Noom's emphasis on social brain research can be especially advantageous for keeping up with long-haul solid propensities. Apps like Headspace and Calm offer guided meditation and relaxation exercises, both of which are important for overall well-being. Mindfulness and stress management are also important. These tools can support your recovery, reduce stress, and improve your mental health. You can effectively manage your recovery after surgery with the help of these websites and apps, which offer a wealth of information and tools to keep you informed, help you make healthier choices and more.

Support Groups and Communities

Support gatherings and networks can play an essential part in your recuperation and long-haul well-being venture. Interfacing with other people who have encountered comparative difficulties offers close-to-home help, useful counsel, and a feeling of the local area. Online care groups, like those found on Facebook and Reddit, offer a stage for sharing encounters, getting clarification on pressing issues, and getting consolation. Facebook groups like the "Gallbladder Removal Support Group" make it safe to talk about post-surgery symptoms, diet changes, and ways to cope. These groups are led by people who have been through similar situations and can provide helpful advice and support.

Numerous support groups, including those devoted to digestive health and problems with the gallbladder, can be found on the website DailyStrength. This stage permits you to interface with others, share your story, and find support from a local area of people who comprehend what you're going through. An opportunity for face-to-face interaction and support is provided by in-person support groups, which are frequently organized by community centers or hospitals in the area. These gatherings are normally driven by medical services experts and deal with an organized climate to examine your recuperation, share tips, and get direction. For those looking for proficient help, working with an enlisted dietitian or nutritionist who has some expertise in post-medical procedure recuperation can be unbelievably gainful. These experts can give customized dietary guidance, assist you with making a fair dinner plan, and proposition progressing support as you conform to your new way of life.

Also, associations like the American Liver Establishment and the American Gastroenterological Affiliation offer assets and backing for people with stomach-related medical problems. Educational materials, support groups, and access to medical professionals who can assist you in your recovery are provided by these organizations. Local area discussions on sites like HealthUnlocked and Motivate additionally offer a space to interface with others, share encounters, and track down help. These discussions are directed to guarantee a protected and deferential climate, and they give an abundance of data from people who have gone through comparative well-being ventures. Taking everything into account, support gatherings and networks give important close-to-home and reasonable help during your post-medical procedure recuperation. Whether on the web or face to face, these gatherings offer a feeling of the local area, understanding, and consolation that can have a massive effect on your journey to better well-being.